The Millenium Diet

The Practical Guide for Rapid Weight Loss

Mark Davis, M.D.

ISBN 978-0-615-20972-2

Library of Congress Number 2008931875

Printed in the United States of America
By Signature Book Printing, www.sbpbooks.com

CONTENTS

FOREWORD

Americans collectively have one of the most unhealthy diets on Earth. With more than 100,000,000 people overweight the logical question to ask is why hasn't anyone in authority or the media acknowledged this health epidemic with more fervor. Or is there another reason why this is not in the forefront of the media daily. The answer to this conundrum though a little unnnerving is obvious. The healthcare industry depends on a constant supply of unhealthy people to keep its infrastructure afloat. This industry as well as the United States government have a vested interest in keeping us as sick as possible. Americans' predilection to ingest unhealthy diets have placed tens of billions of dollars yearly into the coffers of the pharmaceutical, hospital and other industries that support them. Federal and State treasuries are also beneficiaries of this largess. Preventative Medicine is at the very bottom of healthcare expenditures. The Nicotine Industry puts millions of dollars into the pockets of politicians every year. For this reason alone nicotine will never be declared an illicit drug and the millions who succumb to diseases caused by this product will continue to pour into hospitals. Those in the sugar industry are no less guilty. They have invented products such as high fructose corn syrup to rape our pancreases and livers. The results are streams of diabetics seeking medical care for a disease that could be preventable other than for the plethora of sugar that is attacking these organs.

The collective forces at large representing government, the medical profession and private industry pay lip service to any suggestion of improving the contents of our diets. Why should they? Hypertension, hyperlipidemia, high cholesterol and hyperglycemia are caused in large part from our diets and are at epidemic levels. And who benefits from foods fraught with sugar and grease, you guessed it. They do and you don't. The American Healthcare industry has been established to treat people after they incur illness and not before. Have you ever seen anyone from the American Medical Association protesting the contents of cigarrettes. Maybe you have seen documentaries created by the government exposing the food industries' penchant for making some of the most unhealthy products on the planet. Of course not, they don't exist. Unfortunately the story gets more negative. Advertising aimed specifically at children to eat products that are loaded with sugar go unhindered. Have you ever wondered why so many children are labeled ADD or ADHD. Maybe, just maybe its their sugar ridden diets. Half the American population are ingesting pharmaceuticals for many disease states that are preventable. The unabated birth of new medical categorizations to induce more people to ingest drugs is mind boggling. Proper diet is an integral part of the formula for good health and increased longevity. Even the newest gurus of the culinary arts, you know who they are, represent companies that push high glycemic greasy products which will ultimately cause you to partake in the pharmaceutical party that has been going on in the United States for decades.

American dieters have many hurdles to overcome because of the ceaseless propaganda placed in their paths by the food industry to stay heavy. Nutritious advertising is not the lever to sell unhealthy foods. You and I have to be cognizant that the government poorly monitors foods derived from within and outside the borders. We have to take responsibility to choose the correct foods in the proper portions. The Millenium Diet goes back to the basic tenets of food selection. By observation of thousands of patients and their diets over a decade there were certain commonalities that kept them heavy. When these foods were eliminated rapid weight loss occurred. The Millenium Diet has eliminated most of the weight gaining foods and others it has reduced to a minimum. The diet is based on portion control and calories are only used to elucidate certain serving sizes. Calories are cumbersome to deal with and portion control through observation is much easier to learn.

The chapters that follow allow the reader to understand the concepts which have caused them to gain weight and how to completely reverse the trend. Both physiological and psychological aspects of weight gain are covered because at some point they merge to enhance food cravings. Many of the most common questions asked regarding diets, vitamins, exercise and related topics are answered. Successful dieting requires a knowledge of portion sizes. Package labeling is utilized to elucidate nutrient content and serving size. Laws requiring clear package labeling have been on the books for decades. Unfortunately, these laws have been misconstrued so the consumer would get the least benefit from them. The chapter on food labels rectifies this problem enabling the dieter to discern which foods are most appropriate for his or her weight goals. This book contains cutting edge research material and it enhances and expands upon prior texts in this subject area. This book's goal are two fold. One is to inform the reader to rethink the path he or she took while gaining weight. And Secondly, to provide the necessary route to achieve rapid weight loss. The end result is that only through knowledge can your final result be achieved.

INTRODUCTION

Do you want to lose 15 to 30 pounds in the first month of dieting then you have arrived at the correct diet program. There are no gimmicks or pills. No bizarre regimens or ridiculous food products to purchase. This revolutionary diet utilizes normal food products found in your neighborhood grocery to achieve your goal. What is revolutionary about this program is that it has been tested in thousands of patient visits. The patients are the best teachers and with their tremedous input this diet came into being.

Any program that helps achieve a weight loss goal is admirable. We have taken the next step to evolve the diet away from prerequisite recipes or preformed package foods to actually allowing the patient to pick the foods that fit into their lifestyles. The rules within the program are simple and will be covered in the chapters to follow. Dieting is not a one or several day phenomenon. The successful dieter must dedicate him or herself to a program. To many dieters jump to different programs hoping the next one will do the trick. They are only fooling themselves. Losing weight is a very private and personal event in one's life. People arrive at a decision to lose weight for many reasons. Their clothes become tight and a wardrobe awaits their owner's return to their previous weight levels. Some are tired or just do not feel right. For others an event in their personal lives has triggered a return to dieting. Whatever the reason the person becomes aware that something is amiss in their lives and a change is in order.

There are no recipes in this program. There are hundreds of very fine books on the market that give low calorie approaches to preparing meals. Unfortunately, most people do not have the time or inclination to prepare these types of meals. Meal structure defined by portion size is one of the keys to successful weight loss. Once this behavior is learnt losing weight becomes less burdensome to the dieter. Many diets have taught people to withhold one food group over another. The fallacy in this thinking is from the remaining food groups people will simply ingest more. Therefore, the potential to cause weight gain continues unabated. Many programs are not well tested and in the longterm maybe dangerous to your health. The Millenium Diet is well tested, safe and the achievements in many cases are phenomenal.

Why are so many of us overweight has been debated in much of the recent literature. Many dieters will tell you that anxiety led them to over eat. In medical practice this is very common to hear but in a larger frame of reference people simply do not think about how many calories they are eating. Americans have been blessed with an excellent food system from the farm to the grocer to the restaurant. With access to an over abundance of food products people tend not to design meals that are healthy and eat excessive amounts of sugar and fat. The key here is to know exactly what not to eat. Our diet plan will ensure you eat the right foods in the right proportions to lose weight quickly and safely. The small steps people can take in choosing the correct foods and proportions of these items will give them great strides in achieving their weight loss goals.

As alluded to above patients seek out help because they don't feel right. A common statement often heard by healthcare practioners refers to a social or work relationship that soured because of their weight problems. When a person embarks on a weight loss program they are setting out on a very personal journey which is difficult and in many cases frustrating. The format of this diet reduces but does not eliminate these feelings. After a short time the dieter's selection of foods improves dramatically. The external influences to keep their weights elevated diminishes and the process proceeds until the desired weight benefit is achieved.

People often question how did I get this heavy. Statements such as " I was always thin as a child or a teenager" are commonly heard. Weight gain is an accrual process that happens over a period of time. Many people can almost pinpoint the time their weight started to increase. Changing a person's habits is crucial to losing weight but a very difficult process to initiate. The process begins when the prospective dieters are fed up with their weights. By this happening the proverbial one giant leap has occurred. The acknowledgment in their own minds that a change in their lives is in order is the first step. And once this single threshold is crossed the dieter is half way to his or her goal.

Then the question comes about what is the most safe and efficient diet with the most rapid weight loss program. Negotiating the isles at your favorite bookstore one comes upon hundreds of references for weight loss. Everyone has their own formula. This collection of books are written with a flare for the inventive and less for factually based weight loss programs. But they all have one thing one common you must reduce calories in order to achieve sizable weight loss goals. Without considering this first premise of dieting weight loss will not be achieved. So if you are following an all cheese diet or a broccoli and cabbage regimen the bottom line is calorie reduction. Many diets that have no quick weight loss response have had only the most peripheral of testing. Some may even be cardiac toxic. Patients should always check with their physicians if any medical situation precludes them from dieting. Most times a diet will benefit a person that is not in the best health. But only you and your doctor should make those decisions.

Reducing your cholesterol, salt and caffeine will benefit the body greatly and will be advised by all competent healthcare practioners. By following the Millenium Diet the calorie count of the foods you eat will automatically be at reduced levels. The aim of this approach is not only for quick weight loss but to modify your thinking about foods to keep you healthy. Our discussions will start with the precepts of good eating which is embedded into this diet and then discuss the program and how best to utilize its menus with a busy schedule. The major focus of this diet is consistency. The most successful dieter follows the program very closely for best results. Weight reduction is a very private occurrence. Their will be many influences pushing you towards failure. Most will come family and friends. The reasons these people may be a hindrance are many and will be discussed in the chapter on the Psychology of Obesity.

The menus in this book have been used countless times by our patients. Most have achieved major weight loss. Some not at all. The reasons for their lack of success usually comes down to a refusal to change old habits. Choosing appropriate foods is to time consuming and inconvenient for them. Basically, the excuse machine goes into overtime. The patients whose weight loss is minimal to none are counseled intensely. Most come around. Some don't. Usually this small group needs motivation which will develop as the need to lose weight becomes more urgent. They will return when the time is right for them.

The Millenium Diet evolved out of the observations of several thousand patients' dietary habits. Who better to garner information from then the very people who must use the program. Patient feedback was invaluable in building this successful program. Patients from every lifestyle contributed information to derive these menus and we thank them. Before considering dedicating yourself to any weight loss program ask yourself this one question. Is this the most appropriate time for me to initiate a diet? If the answer is yes then you are halfway to the goal line. Once you decide to diet following the program daily is a must. No excuses! If you mess up a meal there is nothing you can do about it but move onto the next one. There are no quick fixes just hard work and dedication with the knowledge that in a short time you will look and feel better.

The Millenium Diet is an excellent road map for rapid weight reduction. It collates the most recent information into one program. All who seek to lose weight will. You now have the latest and perhaps the most original program on the market. Remember the amount of weight loss you will achieve is up to you. So be consistent and focused on the end result. Good luck!

Chapter One

Why Lose Weight

You have now embarked on a major milestone in your life, a weight reduction program. In reviewing what is available to the potential dieter he or she comes across hundreds or perhaps thousands of books on everything from nutrition to food aerobics. The degreed and nondegreed have written books to enable the dieter. The key to every book on the market synergizes down to eating less calories than your body requires. The endless series of ideas concerning weight loss is mind boggling. Good carbs or bad carbs, good fats or bad fats, different types of fiber are all discussed in a thousand variations in these books. Most of these publications may be confusing to the reader and provide peripheral help in the battle of the bulge. There is nothing unique about gaining weight so why should there be about losing weight. People will tell you about specific intervals in their lives when they weighed less. Milestone weights when they were eighteen years old are often heard. Many women will refer to their prepregnancy weight or what they weighed after their last childbirth. References that are usually motivating to get themselves started on a diet. The question most people have is what is the best plan to follow given all the material available. The answer evolved out of thousands of patient visits to our office and is described in detail in the diet chapter.

We know from experience that there is a fade effect that gradually overtakes people who follow most diet programs. That is, the average dieter will be gung ho for a short period of time and follow a diet letter for letter but then lose interest. This time period varies. Reasons most people give for this observation is that the food choices are limited. Some state that their lifestyles preclude them from following a program. But believe it or not many people will tell you that the most inhibitory problem is their family and friends. The subject has come up frequently and many have succumbed to the culinary temptations from those closest to them. The "why" is still elusive. Perhaps these social acquaintances have become conditioned to the idea that weight loss might be equated with poor health. Do you remember the old adage you should eat everything on your plate because there are people in the world who are starving and not as fortunate as us. Early food habits may have evolved from this type of thinking. The clean your plate conditioning maybe manifest in the portions many of us consume as adults. No one knows for sure. But what we overweight people are extremely aware of is weight loss is a must. Depending on what literature you read claims of up to sixty percent of the American society is overweight or obese. With the availability of so much food through our excellent food distribution system it stands to reason that a large percentage of us would become overweight. The process of weight gain by eating more than our bodies require for proper growth starts when we are very young. Many parents start overfeeding their children during their infancy and continue this process not realizing that this practice is nutritionally unsound and could lead their children to become obese adults. Many parents may equate the love of a child with providing an over abundance of food. By gratifying their children with foods laden with sugar the parents are laying out a life long pattern of eating that will result not only in obesity but all the ills that accompany this weight gain. These innate habits fostered over many years maybe the greatest burden the dieter faces.

Why do you want to lose weight? The answer to this question can fill an entire tome of psychology. The realization that your weight somehow hinders you in interactions with your peers. That social acceptance requires a certain look that you do not have. Peer pressure is a major motivating factor in the teenage years. The media displays that all rich and successful stars are thin and have a certain look is all to common. This is a false premise, yet it is presented as true. It is sufficient to state that life long obesity many times has its roots in our youth as noted above and reversing the trend though hard is not impossible. Health reasons are a secondary concern why people come to us for weight loss not primary as one would expect. They are more worried what they look like outside then what ticking time bomb is occurring from within. Fortunately weight loss addresses both issues and most have successful outcomes utilizing the Millenium Diet.

The first thing to consider when starting a new diet is can I dedicate myself to a regimen of lowered calories meaning smaller portions for a specified period of time. If you state at this point you can't then there is no reason to read any further. Never set yourself up for failure by starting something you can't finish. If you state you can then continue reading. Second, you need to push aside any roadblocks that will inhibit your weight reduction program. That is, all the excuses you have been using over the years to continue to eat out of proportion to your physical requirements. Third and final thought before starting your program tell that love one in your life that you plan to lose weight and not to outwardly or subliminally inhibit your goal.

They will know exacly what you mean. By following these three precepts you are already on the road to successful weight loss.

When starting a diet regimen it is important to understand that you have to eat. Those of us who eat sporadically will not lose weight. The most successful dieters understand that they have to eat a minimum of three meals per day. The body has certain rhythms that control food intake, weight gain and loss. These are at the cellular and subcellular levels. Missed meals or minimal intake at a meal will place great physiological stress on these cells that depend on a constant source of nutrients to survive. Internal mechanisms are immediately triggered when the body perceives there has been a prolonged deprivation of food. The body is a lot smarter than people give it credit for by having developed primordial mechanisms to maintain weight in a time of famine. As the lack of food continues the body signals the brain of its increasing hunger. These primodial drives cause the search for food to begin. Luckily, our society has a readily available supply of food. A clear example of the body's innate survival mechanism can be illustrated when deprivation of breakfast occurs. People will over compensate during later meals of the day by indulging their food cravings excessively. Deprivation also slows the basal metabolic rate which makes your body want to hold onto excess body weight longer. Breakfast is an essential meal. Without the primary meal of the day your chances of losing weight are greatly reduced.

When you awake after an extended sleep you may find yourself hungry. Your blood sugar maybe low from not ingesting food for a prolonged period of time. Decreased blood sugar is one of the hints the body uses to encourage you to eat. One must work within the physiology of the body to minimize hunger signals directed at the brain. Eating multiple small meals which includes breakfast allows calories to be spread out through the day preventing overwhelming hunger during any specific time period. Most dieters are under the false impression that skipping breakfast will give them faster results. It is counterproductive for dieter to skip meals because a) you will eat more at a later time negating any of the effects of skipping meals and b) your metabolism may slow in response to extended times without food. Often the patients tell us that they are not breakfast persons. They are too busy to eat the morning meal or the first meal of the day whenever their day starts. But the body knows better and the results are little or no weight loss. I have seen patients who weigh over three hundred pounds tell us they eat like birds.So how does one get that heavy eating like the proverbial bird. The reality is they are eating like eagles but at the wrong times. The excessive intake is usually in the form of carbohydrates which goes unburned by the body and is eventually stored as gross fat. Many people do not wakeup to the fact that their eating habits are so poor that weight gain is inevitable. With dietary modifications and intake of a primary meal the chance of eating more in the latter part of the day is diminished.

Each of us has certain caloric requirements to maintain his/her weight. Below this specific intake one loses weight and above this so called threshhold point weight gain occurs. Calculating the threshhold number is time consuming and has no real value in the realm of weight loss. What is important for us to remember is the set point or threshhold for the number of calories needed to reduce weight is different in each one of us. For the most sedentary person twelve to fourteen hundred calories is in the range that the Millenium Diet aims to provide per day. Enhancements in the diet occurs for specific lifestyles.

For example, running and high intensity athletics requires more calories. As does increased physical labor by virture of the workload requires increased nutritional intake. For the majority of us the twelve to fourteen hundred calorie range will place us in the necessary mode for weight loss.

Examining the type of breakfasts that keep people from losing weight we find that many people consider a cup of coffee a sufficient breakfast. Others consider a nutrient breakfast bar that is sold under many names is enough consumption in the morning. One of the more popular modes is a liquid nutrient supplement either a "power shake" or a canned supplement as the first meal. ALL of these choices are incorrect. Liquids move out of the stomach quickly and release whatever carbohydrates they have in a rapid pace fostering even more hunger several hours later. These modes of eating are setting the dieter up for early defeat and abandonment of their considerations for weight loss. Our goal here is to have you eat a breakfast of sufficient calories and correct content so the hunger is diminished. Foods rich in fiber release their sugars slowly so the body feels satiated longer and cravings for more food comes later not sooner. First lets discuss carbohydrates.

Carbohydrates, the enemy of the American dieter, are complex sugars. The most basic sugar molecule we will be referring to is glucose. Molecules of sugar can bind to each other to form larger entities called starches. Starches will breakdown in the human digestive tract at different rates depending on their chemical and physical makeup. Not all these larger aggregated sugar molecules or starches are the same. Carbohydrates release their sugar products into the bloodstream at different rates. This gives rise to the terms good carb / bad carb. A good carb is one that releases its sugar load more slowly into the bloodstream. Usually the sugars are bound up with fiber in the good carbs causing this delayed sugar release. Some examples of these are fruits, multiple grain breads and vegetables. The so called bad carb releases its sugar content quickly. Some examples of the bad carbs are pastries, white bread and pasta. Much of the fiber has been processed out of these foods. The slowly released sugars tend to be metabolized better and are less often stored by the body. Insulin, a molecule generated in the human pancreas is designed to rapidly clear glucose from the blood. It could either enhance absorption of sugar into a cell where it is metabolized or the molecule of sugar can be stored. Now it gets even more disorienting. Since the bad carbs release their sugar content quickly the body tends to store these sugars and not metabolize them. Those processed foods that release sugars quickly have another downside. As the hormone insulin clears the blood of these sugars hunger returns more quickly then with the unrefined foods we call the good carbs. The premise then is to choose more unrefined foods that have a larger fiber content.

Another concept that needs to be introduced here is that of glycemic index. The glycemic index reflects how fast the body breaks down carbs and the rapidity of blood sugar elevation. The quicker a food elevates your blood sugar the higher the glycemic index. The concept is good to know but the numbers are so variable that some foods are hard to categorize using this term. A carb though is a carb. Meaning it has calories and it has to be burned by the body or it will find its way into storage sites of muscle and fatty tissue. Other concepts such as glycemic load which reflects the amount of starch in a unit of food is a vague term and will not be used here. The rational dieter then will choose foods that have more fiber for breakfast. Power bars, breakfast bars, liquid protein drinks and other contrived foods in these categories will not only stop you from losing weight but may enable your body to gain weight.

We have already established why breakfast is important and we must proceed from this point that following this diet requires you to have a primary meal of the day. Those who have gone down the path of skipping breakfast have learned their weight loss is minimal to none. Eating to few calories during this meal also inhibits weight loss. Consideration should be given to those who do not have the standard nine to five work schedule. If you perform shift work and your day starts at three in the afternoon or eleven at night the three meal day rule still applies. Hunger will not simply abate because you begin work late in the afternoon or at night. People are no less hungry at night than their counterparts on day schedule. These cravings which are driven by the body's ceaselss requirements for sugar are discussed in the next chapter.

Chapter Two

Sweet Tooth

Sugar is the greatest nemesis of the dieter. Sugar derived from sugar cane or beets is utilized in thousands of food products. It comes in many forms including granulated also called regular sugar which is contained in our sugar bowls. Fruit sugar is slightly more fine and is used in gelatins and puddings. It is slightly more uniform in texture than regular sugar. Bakers special is a very fine sugar and is used as the name implies in baking such as cakes, cookies and donuts. Superfine or ultra fine sugar dissolves easily and is used as a sweetener in drinks. Confectioners sugar which has different types depending on the bakers individual needs. Coarse sugar which contains grains that are larger than those of regular sugar are utilized in making liquors. Sanding sugar has larger crystals used in making sprinkles and in baking. There are also a series of brown sugars and liquid sugars used for confectionary purposes. The multiplicity of products containing sweeteners are designed to stimulate both your taste buds and your olfactory sense. The addicting properties of these sweeteners are overwhelming for many of us increasing the challenge for prospective dieters.

Sugar in its most basic form is sucrose. It is a main component of carbohydrates. Sucrose is further broken down by the body into glucose and fructose. These are the most common sugars the body encounters. Lactose which is found in milk products is further broken down by the body into glucose and galactose. To be considered a starch these smaller molecules are connected into larger subunits. Many of our favorite foods can be considered starches such as rice, breads, potatoes and pasta. The body uses glucose for energy purposes and it is the sugar we will refer to when discussing basic carbohydrate metabolism.

It is the sugar molecule that has contributed to the weight gain of tens of millions of people who can be categorized as overweight or obese. Even the government's so called model diet has to many foods with sugar embedded in them. We can't live without sugar. The brain has less than a six minute supply and must continually replenish its sources to survive. Glucose is the body's main source of energy. Scientists state that fifty percent of our diet should come from carbohydrates. The problem is many of us exceed this requirement. Sugar as a source of energy has become the mainstay of the American diet. Unfortunately, if we consume an over abundance of carbohydrates the body will burn only sugar and not fat. If we delete sugar entirely from our diets the body will make it from other sources. This evolutionary mechanism protects our vital organs from any deficits of this molecule. The Millenium Diet adheres to a regimen that requires the dieter to ingest low glycemic index foods in the proper proportion to maximize weight loss.With Americans' proclivity to ingest to many carbohydrates weight gain becomes inevitable. The entire purpose of the diet you are about to embark on is rapid safe weight loss.

Recognizing foods that are high in sugar content are not always easy. Manufacturers have added sugar to thousands of foods far beyond any physiological requirements to ensure your continous repurchase. America is a sugar hustler's heaven. Most packaging labels are written in such esoteric terms it would take a chemistry degree to decipher them. The mere fact that they are written in grams is confusing to people who have been trained in ounces and pounds. Luckily, most manufacturers utilize both systems of measurement. One of my favorite cereal's notes its health benefits on the box. A portion of this cereal without milk is 120 calories. It notes that 28 grams of these 120 calories are carbohydrates. SUGARS!! A gram of either carbs or protein is four calories. A gram of fat is nine calories. Therefore, of the 120 calories, 28 grams times 4 equals 112 are calories deived from carbohydrates. Over ninety percent of this very popular cereal is sugar. The box cleverly draws your attention to its nutritional benefits. Paradoxically, with its enhanced sugar contents and few vitamins added these benefits are nil. Many food labels are deliberately misleading and require futher study. There is an entire chapter devoted to understanding food labels. Minimal health benefits can be derived from foods with high sugar content and knowing the maximum information concerning labeling will be a plus when dieting.

The concept of the glycemic index introduced above is utilized by nutritionists to compare foods. This approach allows someone to understand how the body metabolizes sugars in prospective foods that are chosen. This comparison can be useful in finding the best of the best carbs to eat. Foods with a low index are metabolized more slowly and cause minimal fluctuations in blood sugar. Foods with an elevated index cause major flucuations in blood glucose. Low index diets are fraught with fruits, vegetables and foods with increased fiher content. These type of foods slowly release their sugars and you feel satiated longer. A low glycemic diet is associated with reduced incidence of diabetes, obesity, heart disease and cancer. The calorie structure of many of these foods tends to be less and therefore places less stress on the metabolism. Basically your metabolism does not need to work as hard with this type of diet. The pancreas does not have to supply as much insulin for this low sugar load so your cellular machinery does not need to work overtime to obtain the nutrients from foods. High glycemic index foods typically release their sugars more quickly, have less fiber and are cleared by the blood more rapidly. Some examples of these foods are pasta, pastries and rice. Utilizing the glycemic index as one of a series of references enables us to pick the most nutritious diet for short and long term outcomes. The foods in the Millenium Diet trend towards the lower index group which enhances weight loss and your ability to keep it off.

Examples of some carbohydrates that we recommend are fruits, vegetables, whole grain flour, whole grain cereals, whole grain pasta and legumes, (see menu for portion sizes). The bad carbohydrates are those that have had many of the positive health benefits removed by refining and/or processing. These foods are more tasty but far less nutritious. Many of these foods have preservatives, additives, chemical coloring and flavor enhancements added to their already unnatural states. The body has more difficulty assimilating these categories of foods. The cell structure has to go into overtime to metabolize these foods. Blood sugar is more erratic and satiation is shorter. Some examples of these foods include sodas, pastries, candies and products made with white flour. The enumeration of bad carbs would take an entire book. The important point to remember is these calories have little value in a diet or any health settings. By following the first step in the Millenium Diet which is switching your foods to the essential good carbs that have a low glycemic index your weight will rapidly decrease.

Fructose another sugar has the same chemical formula as glucose but a different molecular structure. It is found in nature in a number of sources including certain vegetables, fruits and honey. Another name for fructose is fruit sugar because it is derived from these products. Fructose is metabolized by the liver and requires no utilization of insulin which sets it apart from glucose which is dependent on this hormone. The benefit of natural fructose is the pancreas gets to rest and insulin remains low. Man has taken fructose to the next level. He enhanced the taste through a series of chemical reactions. High fructose corn syrup is the result. This unnatural sugar is sweeter than its natural counterpart. This chemical is then mixed with glucose in different concentrations before it enters the food chain. In bakery products this artificial fructose may exceed 80% of the total sugar. In sodas it exceeds 50% of the total sugar. Food processors note that high fructose corn syrup is easier to work into their manufacturing schemes and its sweetness is liked by the consumers. What they failed to tell the consumer is this unnatural sugar can cause a fatty liver and elevate levels of blood cholesterol and triglycerides. Most people are unaware of these facts.

With the introduction of high fructose corn syrup in the 1970's the prevalence of obesity in the general population increased to epidemic proportions during the next several decades. By 2002 some estimates have consumption of all varieties of sugar approaching 170 pounds per person per year. Nearly fifteen years earlier it was closer to 120 pounds. Sugar is concealed in so many foods that it was only a matter of time before its effects would show up in the general population. The present epidemic includes over one hundred million people who are overweight or obese. Nearly all of this weight gain has been induced by over consumption of a substance we need little of but crave to a maximum, namely sugar.

Nearly every overweight individual that I have had the priviledge of caring for has presented to our office with a carbohydrate fix or addiction. Each patient would provide a history of nearly uncontrolled desires for sugar laden foods. Pasta, rice, potatoes, white bread and pastries to name just a few items. These foods are not simply used as side dishes to enhance a meal. In many cases they are the meal. Once these foods are ingested the body sees them as sugars. With very few vitamins and heavy doses of sugar these types of foods become very questionable nutrients to sustain good health. Humans no longer eat only for survival. They just eat and eat and eat. As a result all foods once utilized to survive have become instruments of our own demise through their detrimental effects on body's organ systems. With record numbers of people overweight and/ or obese the nation has created a healthcare quagmire that may not be reversible during this present generation. Threaded through thousands of products both at your local grocery and your favorite neighborhood restaurant are foods laden with every conceivable type of sugar the food industry can throw at us. Including but not limited to maltose, dextrose, dextrin, high fructose corn syrup, corn starch, sucrose, fructose and multiple mixtures of the former named sugars. The reason for this explosion of foods full of sugar it keeps you coming back to repurchase more. These very foods are sickening millions of people by destroying pancreatic tissue to cause diabetes and the sundry effects produced by this disease. Diabetes is one of many diseases derived from diets packed with sugar. Vascular and cerebral diseases on an unprecedented scale have been feeding hospitals for the last thirty years. These cases can be counted in the tens of millions. With a budget of tens of billions of dollars health agencies in the Federal government have paid lip service to this problem. The problem is so pervasive using the word epidemic does not do justice to the problem. Since illness is the driving force to keep the healthcare industry's bottom line in the black we never see their representatives publically speaking against those who help feed them, namely the sugar hustlers of America. Therefore, it is up to you to learn what foods not to eat and the Millenium Diet is the perfect vehicle to lead you in that direction.

Chapter Three

The Physiology of Obesity

The human body is not a trash can, yet we utilize it as though it was. Many of us make better selections of foods for our pets than for ourselves. These selections are made by people in all weight classes and are just not reserved for the overweight amongst us. With the evolution of our ability to preserve food through chemistry and refrigeration brought into existence what we now call supermarkets. Thousands of square feet of shelf and refrigeration space devoted to every known food substance on the planet. Many of these processed foods are deleterious to our health, yet they are sold as nutritionally functional products. The success of the food industry's ability to create chemical conglomerations which are sold as borderline food products has displayed the gross failure of the government's monitering programs to keep us safe from these entries into the food chain.

With the introduction of preservatives, chemical "nutrients", food additives, fertilizers, insecticides and radiation of foods our bodies had to adjust to this onslaught of man's proclivity to improve nature. Prior to the discovery of these products food choices were more limited. Yet, the question whether food was more healthy during the prechemical era is answered as a resounding yes! With the rise of many of these so called nutritional derivatives a parallel rise in diabetes, heart disease, hypertension, hyperlipidemia and cancers have been seen in the U.S. population. The human body has not adjusted well to these new food derivatives. The normal mechanisms to clear fats and sugars from the blood stream have either been rendered inefficient or useless. Tens of millions of people are taking lipid reducing drugs, antihypertensive medications, heart and diabetic pills resulting in a large part from the contents of our diets. We are not listening to our bodies when it comes to quantity and quality of foods we are ingesting. The body has very sophisticated mechanisms that control every aspect of the metabolism. It is these mechanisms that have been overcome by these additives and our poor choice of foods. It is very important for those entering into a diet program to have some basic understanding of these mechanisms. The paragraphs below describe many of these systems and how they relate to weight control.

Smoking cessation is a frequent cause of weight gain. The very fear of gaining weight has kept many people from discontinuing this habit. When elevated weight is incurred during nicotine cessation it is usually in the range of five to fifteen pounds. Women tend to gain more than men. The distribution of fat especially in women occurs around the waist. This type of central obesity is associated with an increased incidence of heart disease, stroke and metabolic diseases such as diabetes. Nicotine tends to increase the metabolic rate slightly so a smoker burns more calories than his nonsmoking bretheren. Nicotine works directly on neurotransmitters in the brain to reduce food cravings. In addition to a physiological addiction nicotine also affects the psyche in such a way making withdrawal more difficult. Weight gain can be reduced during the withdrawal phase by utilizing a well constructed diet and nicotine supplements such as the patch or gum. More recently pharmacological agents such as Chantex have been developed which will alleviate withdrawal symptoms and keep weight gain to a minimum. The longterm benefits of smoking cessation offsets any weight gain that maybe incurred. The challenge to controlling weight gain is difficult but many have successfully accomplished this task by perserverence and a well thought out plan such as the Millenium Diet.

Is weight gain a natural part of aging? Most present research indicates that it is. Those who have advanced through the decades will confirm this as a factual statement. Women who are approaching their menopausal years will gain 10 to 15 pounds. They will note an increase in their abdominal girth. As estrogen production decreases from the ovaries the body looks for other sources. Fat cells are capable of manufacturing estrogen. The body will convert its caloric intake into more fat for this purpose. Unfortunately, fat does not burn calories like muscle cells and weight gain occurs. Other hormones in women play a major factor in determining the amount and distribution of their new weight. Men are not exempt from incurring middle age spread. Some of the same hormones effect men's physiology as well. A decline in testosterone which enables the body to create lean muscle mass occurs. The decline occurs in men and to a lesser extent in women. The resulting slower metabolism burns less calories and the inevitable weight gain occurs in both sexes. The good news is that much if not all of this weight gain can be stopped by changing your diet and increasing your exercise pattern. Utilizing weights will allow for much of the lost muscle mass to be rebuilt. Aerobics will help burn any excess calories and is well worth doing. The bottom line is you can avoid much of the consequences of aging by altering a few lifestyle patterns and by not giving in to Father Time.

Most people have heard of the hormone insulin in relation to diabetes. One of its functions is to regulate blood sugar. Another function is to cause sugar to be stored as fat. With the secretion of insulin a cascade of events occurs. Lipoprotein lipase is an enzyme that increases in response to elevated insulin levels. Much of its activities are located in fat cells and blood vessels. As blood sugar increases the storage of it as fat proportionately increases through this enzyme. In reverse, as the body is in diet mode with intake of fewer calories insulin prevents fat catabolism. Insulin also increases triglycerides in the blood stream and enhances protein synthesis. According to present knowledge insulin through its varying interactions with cell structure and lipoprotein lipase will cause the fat content of your body to increase. Insulin is a pivotal hormone in the metabolism of fat. It is one of the hormones the Millenium Diet focuses on.

Sugar and white flour intake have increased by fifty percent in the last twenty five years. The incidence of diabetes has increased proportionally. With excessive sugar intake the pancreas is being shocked with many nutritionally unsound products exhausting this organ's ability to manufacture insulin. The body's insatiable desire for sugar is the direct cause of diabetes in adults. As the pancreas puts out less and less insulin there is a reduced uptake of sugar in the form of glucose by the cells. The level of glucose in the blood stream elevates and numerous negative processes occur over a period of time which makes diabetes a disease to avoid. Those with a genetic propensity for this disease should be especially concerned by their dietary habits. The elevated blood glucose draws fluid out of the cells causing cellular dehydration. The excess fluid takes with it many electrolytes including potassium and other body salts which are excreted with excess volumes of urine. With time there is decreased protein synthesis causing body wasting, vascular degeneration which affects most body organs and reduced immunity. Advanced diabetes is a death sentence and for many of us it is self induced. The body can only utilize a certain amount of sugar to maintain it functions. Diabetes is a result of excess sugar's negative effects on the pancreas. The physiological response resulting from diabetes envelops the body in a cascade of destructive effects which eventually causes death.

Another problem noted with diabetes is insulin resistance. In this condition a sufficient supply of insulin is available but the cells especially fat, muscle and liver utilize it less effectively or are completely unresponsive to its stimulus. The pancreatic response to this resistance is to produce more and more insulin until it eventually exhausts its supply. With this condition blood glucose rises as well as fatty acids. Prediabetes occurs when the blood sugar levels exceed normal limits but are not in the diabetic range. The irony of prediabetes is that simultaneously blood glucose levels as well as insulin levels are high. There maybe tens of millions of prediabetics in the United States. Many of these people will go onto develop type two diabetes which is also called adult onset diabetes. The causes of insulin resistance are many. Since it is frequently seen in families there is a genetic component. Elevated weight levels and lack of exercise contribute to this process. This is not a condition that happens to the other guy. It can happen to you. Those who are persistently heavy over a long period of time have a much greater chance of developing this disease.

The body requires a certain amount of energy to maintain baseline functions. This energy requirement changes as the needs of the body change throughout the day. No two people have the same specific energy needs. There is a fine balance between intake and energy utilization by the body. As the body processes food it utilizes what it needs for energy at that time and stores the rest as glycogen or fat. Evolution has allowed the body to develop mechanisms to store energy. These primordial functions developed because humans did not always have access to food 24/7. These primordial mechanisms have not disappeared. The body does its best to keep itself in a homeostasis. Weight gain is controlled by numerous neural and hormonal mechanisms. Modern man and woman have disrupted the body's control mechanisms by loading up on more food than is required for the body to maintain itself. Weight gain occurs at the point where the burn rate of calories is insufficient to overcome the caloric intake from food.

You can not negotiate with your bodily processes. Many people try to circumvent body physiology by skipping meals, starving themselves for long periods of time, vomiting stomach contents, utilizing drugs to cause accelerated bowel excretions and attempt to speed their metabolisms with medications all in the hope of having a quick weight loss. There are a few short term successes with these approaches but over the long term they are dangerous and will ultimately fail. The body is too smart for these approaches and it will dictate the outcome and not you. The best approach is to work within biologic laws established long before we came into being.

The body has developed counterbalances for every conceivable dietary condition. One of the master hormones as noted above is insulin. The pancreas stores this hormone until it is challenged by a load sugar. Glucagon, another pancreatic hormone comes into play when there is to little glucose in the blood. The mechanism of glucagon is opposite that of insulin. In times of low blood sugar it forces the tissues mainly the liver and muscle to give up glucose that has been stored as glycogen by a process called glycogenolysis. When the supply of stored glucose is reduced the liver can manufacture it in a process called gluconeogenesis. This process enables the body to maintain normal blood glucose in the face of many physiological challenges. Those individuals that eat significantly reduced calories are confronted with these control mechanisms which will maintain homeostasis throughout the body for a limited time until they fail. Many people have been hospitalized because these systems failed at their primary task to keep cellular mechanisms supplied with the energy molecule namely glucose. The challenge for the dieter is to work with these hormonal mechanisms to maximize weight loss. The Millenium Diet performs this function well.

One of the major endocrine glands that controls metabolic activity is the Thyroid. Its activity can induce rapid or slow metabolic responses at the celllular level. The Thyroid gland produces several hormones that controls many aspects of growth and metabolism. When its hormone levels are reduced it could be a cause of weight gain. A child who is born with no or low thyroid hormone may have poor brain development. In adults there are many symptoms of low thyroid hormone. Some of the more common ones are brittle hair, dry skin, slow mentation, low energy levels, cardiac disease, cold intolerance and unfortunately weight gain. The slow onset of weight gain seen in some patients may not key the examining physician into thinking the thyroid could be involved. Many other patients see weight gain in a more acute fashion which elevates suspicion of thyroid deficiency. Women have a higher incidence of thyroid disease then men which should be another indicator for health practioners to be alerted to this disease. With a slower metabolism energy utilization in the body is reduced. The balance between energy utilization and energy intake is then altered. In this scenario more energy is now stored in varying formats. Specifically, as fat and glycogen because the body can not burn all it is consuming therefore weight gain is inevitable.

The typical patient presents to his or her healthcare provider with quasi symptoms. For example, complaining of frequent fatigue or their clothes being tighter than usual. Many of the symptoms delineated in this section on thyroid disease maybe readily apparent to your medical practioner. For confirmation several blood tests are performed which includes a T4 and a TSH. The slow progressive weight gain may abate once thyroid hormone replacement is given. Thyroid deficiency is on is only one link in the algorithm of weight gain so all aspects of this problem should be explored.

Another disease that has challenged the overweight amongst us is called Metabolic Syndrome. This syndrome has five major components. Each component may not always be present but at least three are required to have the syndrome. A waistline of at least 40 inches in the male and 35 inches in the female. An elevated fasting blood sugar over 110. Blood pressure that exceeds 130/85. Triglyceride blood levels that are higher than 150. And the fifth component is a high density lipoprotein (hdl) level in a male of less than 40 and in the female a level less than 50. This syndrome is a prelude to advanced heart and vascular diseases. It indicates diabetes maybe right around the corner. And it sets the stage for a potential terminal event if not addressed quickly and appropriately.

Cortisol, a hormone produced by the adrenal glands, is secreted in response to another hormone in the pituitary gland (ACTH) plays a role in many bodily processes. These include blood glucose regulation, body weight, the immune system, energy balance, the ability to heal physiologically and the ability of cells to become inflamed. Elevated cortisol levels can cause an increase in abdominal girth. Since this hormone is elevated in response to many types of stress it causes the body to give up stored glucose. As blood glucose rises insulin reacts to counter this elevation. Fat formation will occur if cortisol levels remain elevated for an extended period of time. Stress is a key factor driving cortisol levels so high. A reduction in stress will enable the dieter to reduce sugar cravings and hence see a major drop in weight. There is much research in progress concerning stress and weight gain. The answers maybe right around the corner. For now, dieting and exercise are the main avenues for weight loss.

After reviewing some of the internal body processes that can cause weight gain the next section of this chapter deals with a topic of interest to most people. How can humans extend their biological life span? What components of a diet will allow humans to live longer than their present genetic potential permits? More research monies are being applied to this topic because genetics have reached a point where we can now manipulate gene structure to a certain extent. It is only a matter of time before some of the secrets of longevity are discovered.

The ability for an organism to age is a complex relationship that includes but is not limited to nutrition, genetic potential and the environment. At this point in time no one on Earth knows how to extend human life span. Through improvements in healthcare, vaccines, nutrition and improved hygiene we have been able to hold off father time. But we have run up against a physiological barrier to extend life span any further. Studies of animal models are beginning to unveil some of the secrets longevity.

The earthworm has been a fascinating study for scientists for years. With its very short life span, genetic potential and nutrient requirements it is an excellent model to apply longevity research. It is presently known that restricting the caloric intake of the earthworm causes it to live a life span up to three times longer than expected. It not only lives longer but its activity levels parallel those of its much younger counterparts. Its improved viability is not clearly understood but recent studies indicate that certain genes interplay with the changes in nutrition to allow the earthworm prolonged life. As research progresses it maybe possible to determine if certain food restrictions over others are the key to unlock the secrets of its longer life span. The potential to manipulate the specific genes that produce longevity is a major possibility. The obvious question to ask is can longevity studies of the earthworm model apply to humans? The answer is yes.

Humans have a relatively long life span when compared to most animals. Science has already shown that certain restrictive diets can reduce the incidence of heart disease, cancer and diabetes. This allows for a small increase in life expectancy. But is wasn't what the Spanish explorer Ponce de Leon had in mind when he was looking for the Fountain of Youth. In order to apply the studies of lower order animals to humans we would have to study large groups of people for a prolonged periods of time. This is not always feasible because of the long human life span, financial considerations, mobility of the population, differing environments people are drawn from and other factors that make such a study very difficult if not impossible. There are small pockets of people who are attempting to limit their caloric intake to see if their time on Earth can be extended. So far no information has been derived from these groups of people. Unless better methodology appears even designing such a study could be flawed. No one knows whether restricting calories is sufficient or restricting specific food groups is more appropriate. More intriguing is the possibility that certain genes which the changed nutrition would affect could be manipulated to seek the same end point longer life. Pharmacogenetic research may resolve this issue in the next several decades. In this present chapter we displayed how complex the physiology of obesity is. Many of the factors that cause elevated weight can be overcome utilizing appropriate diets such as the one contained in this book. The interaction between our genetic structure and the choices of culinary delights may one day be managed by a pharmaceutical product. Until then losing weight by dieting is the best nonsurgical approach to this widespread problem.

Chapter Four

The Psychology of Obesity

There are many factors that cause us to gain weight. Some are so complex that a textbook in Psychology would be a more appropriate place to discuss these issues. This chapter will review the most common psychological problems related to obesity that healthcare professionals see in their daily practices and how we overcome most but not all of them. Most of the patients that present to our office note they have had a weight problem for years. Many state they feel very uncomfortable discussing weight issues with their healthcare providers. Some have noted that their physicians would avoid discussions of weight control. The sad fact is many patients are under the care of medical professionals on a regular basis yet obesity issues are tangentially discussed.

One third of the American population maybe dieting at any one time. This large number of people represents the depth of the perceived problem in our society. Many people surprisely do not think they are overweight until a health issue related to obesity occurs. Their uncontrolled appetites especially for sugar rich foods are driven by a multitude of issues. For many they call it anxiety eating. Life issues that are so distressing that people take refuge in carbohydrate laden foods. For others they are on auto drive when it comes to choosing foods. There are so many subliminal cues for us to eat the wrong foods that temptation has overwhelmed good thinking. The normal satiation cues are not observed and overeating has become the norm for those without self contained controls.

When a person embarks on a diet he or she should have full understanding why a diet program will be helpful. The specific knowledge of a thorough weight loss program will be useful to set the tone for a behavioral pattern that will be beneficial in the short and the long terms. Whether it is to improve physical stamina or that new look you always wanted it is important to have your minds eye on a reason to lose weight. Once this is established a program of dieting becomes much easier. Unfortunately, many people have already reached the point where their physician has told them to lose weight. Therefore, time will not allow them the luxury of a prolonged diet. Medical problems can not be contained by slow ineffectual diets. The patient's immediate goal should be a well thought out diet plan that can be quickly implemented. The behavioral change required to start such a plan may conflict with the patient's "normal pattern of life"where regimentation such as a weight loss program is a hindrance or interference. TO BAD!! Either you decide to diet or you don't. There is no compromising with your body. A halfway diet is a nondiet and the failure rate is extremely high.

There is no perfect diet. Nothing even comes close. Many people jump from diet program to diet program hoping that the next plan is the one for them. This mind set has caused patients to spend billions of dollars on nonsensical approaches to weight loss finding in the end that they had in their own psyches the ability to lose weight without the trek to the next program. After this self realization that control is within them a concrete pattern of behavior emerges. They realize there is no perfect diet and a clear logical program of restricted food intake is the best approach. Unfortunately for many this realization sometimes comes to late because a medical problem as noted above induced by their obesity has already set in. The approach used here is to prevent the problem before it happens. Preventative medical practices are low on the list of priorities for the medical establishement. No one sees the American Medical Association displaying much concern for the obesity crisis in the country and around the world. The medical establishment garners its income from a continuous supply of unhealthy individuals. Think how many people would be thrown out of work if there were no diseases to care for. Therefore, people must take it upon themselves to prevent disease before it starts.

A question often asked is how long will it take me to lose my weight. Most know the answer before they ask. People lose weight at different rates. Their sense of urgency is out of proportion to the enormous weight loads they have accumulated over many years. That is, the quick weight loss mode they are searching for can not occur because of the physiological barriers that are innnate to human genetics. People place unreasonable time limits on their diet programs. Many times the patients are surprised how fast they lose when they follow a methodical program. No one knows better than the dieter all the pitfalls and inhibitions that make losing weight a nonlinear process. For many there are tremedous psychological barriers to overcome before starting any regimented diet program. Research noted below discusses many categorizations of emotional eating.

Doctor Roger Gould, M.D., psychiatrist, author and lecturer delineates in his writings on the subject of diet the many facets of emotional hunger. In his research he notes dieters have twelve types of emotional hunger to overcome. These intuitive categorizations become obvious when dealing with dieters who have a multiplicity of reasons for gaining weight. They correctly describe many of the inhibitions people use as an excuse not to lose weight.

Type 1

He notes if you get angry, anxious, bored or lonely you suffer from type one emotional hunger and food is utilized to dull the pain derived from these emotions. A common problem and one the patients will not readily relate to you. As they feel more comfortable with the diet therapist these problems become more evident. A percentage of patients are taking various antiaxiety drugs or antidepressants. Even with these drugs many people can not reconcile these problems totally and other interactions are required.

Type 2

Someone who feels belittled, taken advantage of or talked down to eats to avoid confrontation. Many patients who have expressed this type of situational problem were conflicted at work or home by a boss or a spouse who was confrontative in nature and looked for solace in food. Food is their analgesic and the ensuing weight gain is the result.

Type 3

Craving food may occur when you have tensions with a close relationship. Eating is utilized to avoid the pain of rejection or anger. Commonly seen especially in our female patients. The patient internalize this type of problem and food softens the impact of these emotions.

Type 4

If you are overly critical of yourself or think you are less than others around you then this categorization maybe what causes you to overeat. You may think of yourself as a loser, stupid or just lazy. These feelings are the driving force behind this type of overeating.

Type 5

Your hunger may increase because you have less than a satisfactory intimate relationship with your close companion. This failure is reflected in the lack of trust or feeling of insecurity in your emotional union. The driving force behind your hunger maybe the anxiety induced by this perceived failed relationship.

Type 6

Deprivation you experienced as a child may cause you to emotionally eat. This could have been manifested by having a very critical parent. Perhaps a parent who was detached from you and rarely displayed any affection for you. Or one that was physically abusive. Also in this category is poverty and all the misery incurred by it.

Type 7

If you overeat to assert your independence to display you are in control of your life this category describes your situation. I have seen this behavior displayed in teenagers but it is not isolated to this group. Many newly separated or divorced individuals will display this type of behavior.

Type 8

Appetite increases when a person is faced with new challenges. Dr. Gould describes food being utilized to avoid rising to the new task presented. Food is used to insulate oneself from failure. A new workplace or entering college are some situations where this behavior maybe found.

Type 9

A very common reason people stay overweight is to reduce their attractiveness so no one would desire them for sexual encounters. Some of the most attractive people have allowed their weights to balloon because of failed sexual relationships. Most of the people in this category share issues with some of the other types.

Type 10

This type of overeater intakes more food than required as a payback for someone hurting them in the distant past. Within this distorted thinking the person works out their resentments by utilizing their body perhaps by disfiguring it in an attempt to get even with the other party who caused the "hurt".

Type 11

Some people eat to make themselves carefree as though they are still children. This type of eating may help them cope with the challenges of growing up. Many people do not want to face the realities and responsibilities of adulthood. These adult children for lack of a better term are the Peter Pans of their generation.

Type 12

The last of Dr. Roger Gould's emotional hunger delineations is the fear of getting thin whether consciously or subconsciously. Very few of my patients have exhibited this behavior. The cases that I have seen are people from families that are generally heavy. The social influences to stay heavy are ever present.The two examples below will illustrate this type of emotional eating.

Patient A, is a thirty year old female who lost forty pounds. Her husband observing her rapid weight loss over several months became irate at her and the healthcare provider, this author. The husband accused our office of making his wife sick but in actuality she looked more youthful and attractive. He felt threatened at his wife's new appearance. She did not visit the office for several months and in that interim she regained her lost weight and more.

Patient B, was a twenty year old male who weighed 300 pounds with a height of six foot and one inch. He worked nights as a security guard. He was loosing weight steadily over a ten week period. On his third visit to our office he brought with him his mother and grandmother. They were both appalled at his restricted caloric diet. The comments from these two family members were less than friendly. I explained the methodology and the reasoning why this diet causes rapid weight loss. He never returned after this visit. Their innate fear of him losing weight when they kept him heavy through childhood may have been a protective mechanism open to your own interpretaion.

Categorizations such as the Twelve Emotional Hungers by Dr. Roger Gould help us to achieve greater weight loss results by understanding why people gain weight in the first place. Major depression after emotional trauma is a frequent reason for weight gain and many of the fine commercially available diet programs are not set up to deal with these type of patients. The natural tendency for most of us to grab for highly carbohydrate laden foods is multiplied many times by those with emotional traumas. The hundreds of stories that can be related to illustrate emotional traumas causing weight gain would go beyond the scope of this book. But understanding them helps those who have been thin and gained substantial weight return to previous weight levels prior to their personal traumas.

One of the most interesting research papers recently published (The Spread of Obesity in a Large Social Network over 32 Years by Nicolas A. Christakis, M.D., Ph.D., M.P.H. and James Fowler, Ph.D., in the New England Journal of Medicine, July 26, 2007) was an analysis of medical records from the Framingham Heart study following residents of a Boston suburb for thirty two years. The findings confirmed what many of of us suspected that within social relationships obesity is contagious. Social ties appear to have a stronger relationship in causing weight gain than what is evident in our present knowledge of genetics and obesity. The study found a person's chances of becoming overweight or obese increased by 57% if a friend became obese, 40% if a sibling became obese and 37% if a spouse did. The authors note that the closest relationships increased the risk of becoming obese by a factor of three. Some of the thoughts expressed in their research paper note that by having relatives and friends who are overweight or obese one's idea of acceptable weight changes. They also noted that gender relationships had a strong influence on weight gain. The risk between brothers and/or sisters increased dramatically. This study was limited to a suburb of Boston but the information is a useful tool to gain insight in weight gains in relationships.

Researchers James O. Prochaska and Carlo DiClemente (Changing for Good, 1992, published by William Morrow) have identified six stages of behavioral change that are utilizable as a model in weight management. Precontemplation, Contemplation, preparation and determination, action, maintenance and termination. In each stage the patient's thinking is the key to successful weight loss.

1) Precontemplation: A patient may not be aware he or she has a weight problem. The patient sees no need to diet, exercise or change lifestyle habits. Some may not be interested in weight loss and refuse to discuss it.

2) Contemplation: The patient considers the risks and benefits of changing weight behavior and is waiting for the right momemt to begin diet and exercise. They wish the problem behavior would resolve itself.

3) Preparation and Determination: The patient plans to initiate weight behavior change and is motivated and ready to learn about diet and exercise.

4) Action: The patient has achieved consistency with changed weight behavior, weight loss is visible and he/she is confident about maintaining the change.

5) Maintenance: The patient has incorporated new weight behavior in his or her daily life, avoids backsliding and is confident concerning continuing the changed diet behavior.

6) Termination: Patient has continued his/her new behavior for over one year, has avoided relapses and is confident that the new diet behavior will continue.

The authors of the Behavior Change Model were ingenious in defining the stages that most of us who diet move through which enables the medical practioner to provide appropriate intervention at the proper level. Many people have moved through these steps multiple times in their lives. The imperfect nature of all efforts to diet occurs because of the human element. No one follows any program absolutely and this research allows for more practical thinking when dealing with dietary issues. With this in mind the attempt to categorize eating habits is the best tool we have to provide appropriate intervention.

Two of the most frequent psychological conditions encountered by medical personal during weight control intervention are anxiety and depression. In our practice nearly one in four patients are taking medications to improve mood and outlook. All were diagnosed by their primary care physicians utilizing very different criteria to begin these drugs. Many patients are diagnosed incorrectly and the drugs they are using have very little effect. Many people who present for weight loss therapy have had short episodes of anxiety but were placed on longterm therapies. The crutch of an incorrect psychological diagnosis may inhibit the patient's efforts to lose weight because it is this diagnosis that has caused the initial weight increase. The following example will illustrate reasons why proper psychological diagnoses are a must and standards should be appropriately considered before medications are prescribed.

Patient C is a twenty four year old female whose weight had ballooned to three hundred pounds over a four year period from an initial weight of one hundred forty pounds. Several failed relationships have caused her to live a near reclusive existence. She lives alone alienated from most of her family. Her emotions drove her to eat unchecked and by the time she sought help her weight had doubled and her anxiety had turned into a deep depression. This scenario is more common than one would think. She needed psychological care and immediate weight loss intervention. By the very fact she was seeking help she had worked through the first several stages of the Behavioral Change Model that she was determined to lose weight. Unfortunately, her primary care physician told her to exercise and reduce her carbohydrate intake without exploring the real problem she had which was depression. Her weight gain continued until her she was properly diagnosed and today her weight is down nearly twenty five percent from her presenting weight and she is in new relationship.

Anxiety and depression caused by day to day stresses of life have driven tens of millions of people to take medications to remedy these perceived psychological ills. The range of psychiatric complaints includes very mild emotional symptoms to deep depression. One of the most frequent signs of mental distress is weight gain. Each individual who has presented to us has a unique story how his or her weight increased following a mental trauma. Some people can not remember when and why their weight increased. Many diet programs fail to understand that even if the appropriate categories of food are chosen many people will continue to consume excess amounts. In order to successfully lose weight one must not only be placed on a restricted diet, one must understand that mental discipline is the most important element of a successful weight loss program. Most of the patients overcome these concerns by regimentally preplanning their meals. Those patients whose anxieties drive them beyond their abilities to cope with limited food intake are treated by their primary care physicians with medications to resolve these issues first.

In a study by the National Institute of Mental Health published in the Archives of General Psychiatry, July 2006 edition, noted that one out of four cases of obesity is associated with anxiety or mood disorders. The exact nature of this relationship was not clarified by this study. The study was based on a survey of 9282 adults from the United States. These results note that a rise in obesity in America is associated with increasing rates of depression, bipolar disorders, panic disorders and other psychiatric conditions. This study found no difference in the rates between men and women as other studies have found. Another very interesting finding noted obesity was associated with a 25% lower risk of having a substance abuse disorder. The casual relationship between these disorders and obesity are continuing to be defined. Diet plans will need to be adjusted as new confirmatory data is derived. The important point to remember is early intervention by a properly trained healthcare professional can resolve many of the psychiatric causes of obesity.

Chapter 5

The Diet

When your eyes look at food it sees a distinct entity such as a plate of spaghetti or a slice of pizza. What your metabolism sees once you ingest these foods are protein, sugar and fat the essential components of all food groups. The body can synthesize all the sugar it needs without having to ingest any. Fat and protein must be eaten to maintain life functions. The body has had millions of years to develop systems to utilize these food groups to preserve life. In a few short generations humans have developed processed foods that counter genetic history to cause death from the very substances that are supposed to sustain us. Collectively, Americans are a very unhealthy society caused in great part from its food supply. To reverse a very serious trend where one hundred million people are weight challenged is a task that can be overcome by a very sensible approach. Since most people have not learned proper eating habits the school system can and should give courses in nutrition. Starting in the elementary years schools should begin discussing nutritional issues and how they relate to our health. Proper eating is a learnt behavior like any other and should be treated in a similar fashion. Many obese kids come from families where their parents are also obese. This correlation is undeniable. Many behaviors need to be unlearned. The school systems' ability to reach tens of millions of children early in their lives can make a great impact on their nutritional thinking. The diet enumerated below integrates solid thinking into its design and those educated to it benefit both by improved health and rapid weight loss. The diet was created around a core of appropriate protein, carbohydrate and fat combinations which allow for enhanced weight loss with foods commonly available. Weight loss up to thirty pounds in under six weeks has been achieved utilizing this diet model. Those who applied all facets of the diet program had the best results. The well tested menus below were utilized by our patients to achieve maximum results. The portions below are restricted in such a manner to help burn fat and for safe expedited weight loss.

You must choose only the food products on the lists or any types that are similar in nature. Remember to be very successful you must chose the proper foods in the appropriate amounts to achieve the greatest results. The menus are self explanatory. The lists entitled do or do nots below each meal apply not only to the meal titled above it but also to the other meals throughout the day. Major deviations from the menus and the food lists will inhibit your success. Please adhere to them carefully and you will be pleasantly surprised how your weight diminishes very rapidly.

Breakfast Menus

Menu 1

1 choice from the fruit list with a choice of either of the following:
½ bowel of cereal from list with 4 to 6 ounces of skim or 1% milk

or

1 whole wheat bagel or 1 whole wheat English muffin.

Menu 2

2 Egg Beater eggs or equivalent
2 pieces of thin sliced whole wheat bread
1 piece of fruit from the list

Menu 3

2 fruits from the list plus one yogurt (120 calories plain or with fruit)

or

3 pieces of fruit from the list

Menu 4

4 to 6 ounces of 2% cottage cheese
2 pieces of fruit from the list

Menu 5

Vegetable egg omellete (2 eggs plus vegetable choices)
2 pieces of whole wheat bread or 1 whole wheat bagel or 1 whole wheat English mufffin

Do Nots List

No cereals with added sugar

No peanut butter

No cream cheese this includes the dietetic versions

No power bars

No breakfast bars

No nutrient bars

No commercial breakfast drinks

No regular jelly

No fruit juice (see exceptions on do list)

No soy milk

No white bread

No white rolls or equivalents

No pastries

No butter or margerine (see exceptions on the do list)

No pancakes, waffles or French toast

No maple syrup, no corn derived syrups nor honey, no white or brown sugar

No cheese

Absolutely no convenience foods from your favorite fast food chains

No potatoes for breakfast

Do List

A) Cereals

1) Total with or without fruit

2) Special K with or without fruit

3) Plain oatmeal

4) Rice Crispes

5) Kashi

6) Raisin Bran

7) Any equivalent cereal without added sugar or nuts

B) Milk a) skim, b) 1%, c) lactase free skim or 1%

C) Spray margarines which contain no calories, light quantity recommended

D) Sweet and Low, Splenda, Neutra Sweet, Equal or no calorie equivalents

E) 1) No more than six large eggs in any one week or

2) Egg Beaters or equivalent instead of regular eggs, 2 eggs per day

F) 1) 100% whole wheat bread

2) 100% whole grain bread

3) whole wheat bagel

4) whole wheat English muffin

G) Pam or no calorie equivalent for frying

H) Four to six ounces of orange juice for breakfast only

J) Vegetable omelette= 2 egg equivalents with tomato, onions etc., or other vegetable choices

Lunch Menus

Menu 1

A salad consisting of 1/3 to 1/2 head of lettuce, tomato (medium, approxmately five ounces), Celery, cucumbers, onions and carrots. No croutons or bacon. A light amount of parmesan but no other cheese. Four ounces of chicken, not fried, permitted. Dressings see list.

Menu 2

2 slices of 100% whole wheat bread
Fish or meat choice, approximately 4 ounces
Plain mustard or a diet version of mayonaise
Lettuce, tomato and onion
1 piece of fruit

Menu 3

Fruit platter choice= 3 to 4 fruits from list
4 ounces of 2% cottage cheese or a yogurt (approximately 120

calories
plain or with fruit)

Menu 4

Prepared commercial meals of approximately 350 to 400 calories.
These meals should contain preferably chicken or fish. Find meals without gravy, cheese or bread.
Menu 5

4 to 6 ounces of chicken, baked or broiled
2 vegetable choices, 1 fruit choice

Menu 6

Steamed vegetable platter (3 to 4 vegetables from list)
4 to 6 ounces chicken or fish, baked or broiled

Menu 7

Vegetable soup or light consomme approximately 6 ounces
2 pieces whole wheat bread
1 piece of fruit from the list
4 ounces of chicken or fish

DO NOTS

1) No cheese except parmesan sprinkled on your salad

2) No bread, rolls, subs, baguettes or bagels made with white flour

3) No pastries

4) No regular mayonaise

5) No ketchup

6) No mixed meats such as spam, bologna, hot dogs or liverwurst

7) No bacon

8) No fast/convenience foods from your favorite sites

9) No chips of any kind or nuts

10) No pizza

11) No fried foods

12) No creamy or thick soups

13) No soups containing wontons, potatoes or heavy broths

14) No canned fruits or vegetables

15) No crab cakes

16) No oils on your salad

17) Do not fry any foods in oil

<u>DO LIST</u>

1) Fat free or low calorie salad dressings use only two tablespoons which is the equivalent of 1 ounce. Total calories should not exceed 60.

2) Plain mustards only

3) Light mayonaise used judiciously on your bread or mixed with your favorite food

4) Only fresh or frozen fruits and vegetables

5) 4 to 6 ounces of meat preferably chicken or turkey. Red meats should be the leanest you can find within this portion size. There are several varieties of very lean ham that are excellant supplements to a diet but do not consume any other pork products. Cold cuts are also acceptable including chicken, turkey, lean ham or lean roast beef.

6) Most fish are acceptable in the 4 to 6 ounce range. Tuna in water is an excellant choice with your lunch.

Acceptable Drinks

1) Water is your best friend on a diet. Please drink as your needs dictate. There is no reason to over ingest fluids. Flavored waters are accpetable as long as the serving size is less than ten calories.

2) Soda should have no calories and preferably without caffeine

3) Crystal Lite

4) Ice tea with sugar substitute

5) Coffee, preferably low caffeine, nondairy creamer or 1% milk, sugar substitute

6) Green Teas with sugar substitute

7) Milk, skim or 1%

Unacceptable Drinks

1) Energy drinks

2) Sugared sodas

3) Fruit juices, except 6 ounces of orange juice for breakfast

4) Alcohol in all forms

5) Regular milk (whole milk)

6) Chocolate milk

7) Soy milk

8) Milk shakes or ice cream sodas

9) Fruit drinks made with sugared syrups

Dinner Menus

Menu 1

4 to 6 ounces of meat from the list

2 choices of vegetables from the list
1 carb choice from list

Menu 2

4 to 6 ounces of fish from the list
2 vegetable choices from the list
1 carb choice from the list

Menu 3

Vegetable platter with 4 choices from the list
2 pieces of whole wheat bread or 1 carb choice

Menu 4

Fruit platter with 4 choices from the list
4 to 6 ounces of yogurt or 2% cottage cheese

Menu 5

Restaurant food is acceptable as long as it conforms to the food lists and portion sizes within these present menus.

Meat and Fish choices

1) 4 to 6 ounces of chicken, baked or broiled

2) 4 to 6 ounces of turkey, baked or broiled

3) 4 to 6 ounces of very lean red meat, grilled or broiled, When frying red meat use a noncaloric agent such a Pam

4) 4 to 6 ounces of fish chosen from the following list, baked or broiled. It should never be cooked in oil or grease.

    a) Tuna packed in water

    b) Cod

    c) Halibut

    d) Salmon

    e) Shrimp

    f) Crab

    e) lobster

Dinner Carbohydrate list

1) Rice, ½ cup (precooked) preferably brown

2) Pasta, ½ cup (precooked) whole grain preferably

3) One average size potato no more than twice a week. The potato should never be fried nor should you add cheese, butter or sour cream. A sweet potato of similar size maybe substituted (do not add any glazes or toppings to it).

Fruit List

Portion size: One medium or one cup

1) Orange

2) Grapefruit

3) Tangerine

4) Tangelo

5) Apple

6) Pear

7) Apricot

8) Peach

9) Cantaloupe

10) Watermelon

11) Blueberries

12) Strawberries

13) Nectarine

14) Medium Banana

16) Grapes, red or green, 16 to 20

<u>Vegetable</u>

Portion size: One cup

1) Asparagus

2) Broccoli

3) Brussel sprouts

4) Cabbage

5) Celery

6) Carrots

7) Cucumbers

8) Eggplant

9) Green beans

10) Lettuce

11) Mushrooms

12) Okra

13) Onions

14) Peas

15) Peppers

16) Radishes

17) Spinach

18) Squash

19) Tomato (defined as a fruit but is used as a vegetable)

20) Turnips

21) Zucchini

Avoid fish products such as crab cakes which have multiple ingredients and are not desirous for dieting. There are many excellent recipes for fish. Unfortunately, they add butter, mayonaise and white flour. During a dieting period it would be better to avoid these recipes.

Rice comes in numerous varieties. Recommended most is brown rice because it retains its nutrient value. If you prefer only white rice no more than ½ cup (precooked). As a side dish rice works well to supplement a dinner and your carb cravings.

Pasta also comes in numerous categories recommended most is whole grain. No more than ½ cup dry, precooked, with your meal.

Potatoes, no more than twice a week (medium size). The potato skin is the most nutritious part. The rest of the potato your metabolism sees as a sugar derivative and will cause weight gain. Avoid french fries and other potato formats. Do not use sour cream, cheese or any other high calorie additions.

This is a normal salt and spice diet. Consult with your doctor if a health problem prevents you from utilizing these ingredients.

Soy proteins have recently become very controversial because the isoflavones contained within them have mild estrogenic properties that have been linked to cancers in women. This is not a conclusive fact so the controversy persists. Soy protein contains all the amino acids the human body requires to perform its functions. The substitution for soy protein over animal protein has the added benefit of not having saturated fats embedded in it. Though soy protein may have positive cardiac benefits many of the foods using soy products do not fit into regimens created for this diet. I request the dieter who wants to take full advantage of this program not to use soy products until he or she gets to their desired weight.

Do Nots

a) No gravies

b) No cheese or cheese sauces

c) No white flour based products

d) No pizza

e) No chinese food except steamed vegetables supplemented with either steamed chicken or steamed shrimp.

f) No crab cakes

g) No ketchup

h) No tacos or equivalent

Evening Snack

For those who want an evening snack the following list has been utilized successfully in the course of a rapid weight loss program. Choose one from the list. Do not ingest a snack within two to three hours of sleep.

1) ½ cup of cereal choice with skim or 1% milk

2) ½ sandwich (100% whole wheat) with 2 ounces of meat/fish

3) 1 fruit choice

4) 2 cups light popcorn without butter

5) 1 serving size of whole wheat pretzels

6) 1 serving size low-cal jello or low-cal pudding
   (These are the kind you have to prepare)

7) Crystal Lite icepops or equivalent (absolutely no ice cream of any kind)

Do Nots for Snacks

1) No nuts of any kind

2) No potato chips or equivalent

3) No buttered popcorn, no movie style popcorn

4) No cheese doodles, cheese balls or equivalent

5) No pastries

Chapter Six

Common Questions asked by Dieters

Q) What is the best exercise to enhance weight loss?

A) An aerobic exercise will enable the quickest weight loss. There is no one specific best aerobic exercise. Most literature on exercise physiology recommends a quick paced walk to a jog. Approximate distance of two miles three days per week as a minimum. This will increase your basal metabolic rate so calories will be burned at an enhanced rate long after the workout is completed. Any aerobic exercise done for at least thirty minutes three times a week will be a big plus in the weight loss equation for the dieter. Toning exercises such as resistance training with weights over the long term will increase muscle mass subsequently improving the body's ability to burn calories. Therefore, both types of exercise over the long term will enhance weight loss.

Q) What are the best vitamin and mineral supplements to use?

A) Vitamins and minerals are nutrients that the body requires to perform its essential functions. Most multiple vitamins are built around a certain fixed model which contain the recommended dosages of all key vitamins and minerals. The numerous choices on the market use this fixed model. Whether purchasing a brand name or an off brand most are made by a few companies and comparative shopping will note the ingredients in these supplements look just about the same. The best choice is one that contains both vitamins and minerals without herbal products. Herbs do not serve as required nutrients and therefore are not needed by the body. If you have a requirement for a specific herbal substance then purchase it separately. Chances are there is only a trace amount in the vitamin supplement. Some brands to compare are Centrum, GNC Ultra Mega Formulas and Kirkland.

Q) What if I don't feel like eating should I still eat three meals a day?

A) The answer is a resounding yes especially when dieting. The body requires a certain amount of nutrients to survive. Our metabolism burns food at a specific rate while we are sedentary. By presenting to many calories to it at any one time the body will store the breakdown products of food until they are needed. Eating the right type of food and slightly less than the body requires, the metabolism will draw energy from stored body materials namely fat, therefore weight loss occurs.

Q) What is the difference between trans fat and cis fat? Also the significant differences between saturated and unsaturated fat.

A) Trans and cis fatty acids are molecular isomers of each other. This means they are mirror images of each other which contain the same exact constituents but are arranged differently. Trans type fats have been found to be toxic to the heart and should be avoided. The cis variety has not. Saturated fats are substances that the body has more difficulty metabolizing than unsaturated fats due to the chemical nature of their bonding. For health purposes try to avoid saturated fats because they will accumulate faster in the vascular tree especially around the heart. For weight loss purposes all fat should be kept to a minimum because of their high caloric content. We recommend 30 to 35 grams of fat per day, 80% to 90% should be unsaturated in nature.

Q) What is the latest time I should eat prior to sleep?

A) We know that during sleep metabolism continues to work burning calories. When too many carbohydrates are presented to the body prior to sleep insulin levels will increase and the body will continue to burn these carbs over fat during sleep. By having a light snack including but not limited to a fruit, vegetable or a low carb product the body will keep insulin levels low and allow fat catabolism to occur. Insulin does not only control sugar metabolism it is the pivotal enzyme in fat storage and breakdown. Lower insulin levels allow fat breakdown. Therefore, the late night snack should be low in carbs and should not be ingested within two to three hours of sleep. This will allow the stomach to empty and the insulin surge that occurs to metabolize the small amount of sugar ingested.

Q) What is the best diet available?

A) There is no one best diet. The present diet contained in this book includes the the latest research for quick safe weight loss. Many diet programs take advantage of a certain food group, quantity of that food or both. The best science presently available directs us to utilize the following premises: a) you must want to lose weight, b) portion control is a must, c) an elevated protein diet with a moderate amount of carbs and low fat will increase the rapidity of weight loss. Since the body has the capacity to make all the sugar it needs a diet lower in carbohydrates will not affect a person's health and will allow the body to shift into a fat burning mode instead of one that utilizes only sugar. Many dietary programs cause a slow loss of poundage because they do not take full advantage of the human metabolism. They provide too many poor quality carbohydrates which inhibit the body from burning fat. Many dieters do not mind losing two to four pounds per month. Others are looking for a much quicker weight loss. The value of a lower carbohydrate diet allows the body to gear up its metabolism towards fat burning and such a metabolism can lose weight many times the weight loss represented by the higher carb programs. Our unique metabolism basically dictates the lowered carb approach as the optimum program that science can offer us presently.

Q) What is the best time to exercise?

A) There is no best time to exercise. Logical thinking dictates that when one is least tired the most efficient and productive exercise occurs. Late day fatigue might be an inhibitory factor for exercise. Yet, millions of people exercise in the evening without detriment. There are no studies to validate a best time to exercise. The best answer is exercise when you are least fatigued and the exercise time will be used more effectively.

Q) How many carbohydrates should I ingest in twenty four hours?

A) There is no single answer that fits here. In a review of the last ten diet books printed each author states his or her own conception of total carb intake for twenty four hours. Even nutritional scientists vary on the quantity of carbs a person should ingest during this time period. Many believe that fifty percent of your intake should carbohydrates. The Mellenium Diet is forty to fifty percent carbs. The important point to remember is the correct type of carbs should be ingested as noted in the menus. Those with low glycemic indices that is foods that do not cause large amounts of sugar to be absorbed quickly are preferred. Please see diet selections.

Q) How much fluid should I drink?

A) The human body loses water through a number of mechanisms including perspiration, urination, respiration and bowel functions. In addition, the environment plays a key role in fluid requirements. Approximately sixty percent of the adult body is composed of water. Every system in the body requires fluid replenishment. Fluid intake should be approximately 2.5 liters for women and 3 liters for men daily. Which means approximately 9 to 10 cups for females and 13 to 14 cups for men. Humid environments and exercise increase fluid requirements as does certain disease states. As food is processed in the gut the supply of fluids present enhances absorption. So staying well hydrated is a plus for weight loss. Two factors to keep in mind are low or no calorie drinks are preferred when dieting and over hydrating might be dangerous and will not enhance your final weight loss goals. Don't forget that many foods including fruits and vegetables provide fluid to your body and should be part of the over all equation of fluid intake.

Q) How many calories should I ingest in a 24 hour period to lose weight?

A) This is the million dollar question. Nearly every diet book author and nutrition scientist agree to disagree on this point. Two factors that have an immediate impact on the amount of calories the body requires are human activity levels and basal metabolic rate. More active individuals have increased caloric requirements. Those with a more sedentary nature require less. The concept of basal metabolic rate concerns how the body utilizes energy. It is the burn rate of calories by someone who is sedentary throughout a twenty four hour period. Remember you burn calories whether asleep or awake. The basal metabolic rate slows as we age. It will slow if you deprive yourself of a meal or meals in the hope of losing weight faster. Utilizing this information and learning from the experiences of thousands of patients, a diet consisting of twelve to fourteen hundred calories appears to be the optimum calorie count to effectuate weight loss. Those with heavier expenditures of energy through work or exercise should adjust their diets to meet these additional demands. Remembers the old premise if you take in more than you metabolize your weight will increase and the converse is also true weight loss will occur when food intake is less than energy expenditure.

Q) Why can't I skip breakfast?

A) Breakfast maybe the most important meal of the day for a number of reasons. When you wake up in the morning your blood sugar is low (unless you made a quick trip to the refrig. in the middle of the night). With a low blood sugar your body will usually crave food unless you are one of the millions of people who have learned to skip breakfast thinking you will lose weight faster, which is not the case. The delayed intake of food in the morning may slow your metabolism and secondarily cause you to crave more food later in the day to over compensate for the lost calories. Eating breakfast will cause your metabolism to jump start providing needed energy to initiate many bodily systems. Specifically, insulin levels and the cascade of enzymes it initiates will function more efficiently helping the cells to burn the current food intake. People who eat breakfast find their weight loss improves because they spread the caloric intake throughout the day and do not overload the metabolism at anyone specific meal.

Q) How can alcohol affect my diet?

A) Alcohol will increase weight by providing additional calories to your metabolism. The sugars created will place additional stress on a number of systems including your liver and pancreas. Your pancreas will produce more insulin which will eventually cause fat deposition. In the liver ketones will be formed from alcohol preventing fat breakdown from occurring. During a reduced calorie diet the body burns fat as ketones. Alcohol then becomes the source of ketone production instead of your fat. You stay heavy.

Q) What is the meaning of glycemic index?

A) The glycemic index denotes how fast a given carbohydrate is processed by the body and enters the blood stream as compared to glucose. Carbohydrates with a lower glycemic index enter the blood stream more slowly. Those with a higher index enter more quickly. For dieters the lower glycemic index foods will accelerate weight loss. Fruits and vegetables have a lower index. Foods made with white flour have a higher index.

Q) What are ketones and how are they involved with weight control?

A) Ketones are products of fat catabolism. When the intake of carbohydrates is restricted insulin levels are reduced and the body changes from a sugar burning mode to a fat burning one. Ketones are mildly acidic body byproducts which are a type of reserve fuel when carbohydrates are restricted. Ketones can inhibit the release of insulin from the pancreas. Therefore, blood sugar becomes more even and reduces food cravings.

Q) What is a ketogenic diet?

A) Diets that are low in carbohydrates which depend on ketosis for weight loss are designated ketogenic diets. Those who have liver, kidney or other metabolic conditions should not utilize a ketogenic mode of dieting.

Q) Can someone eat to much healthy food?

A) Yes, because a food is considered healthy does not mean it has reduced calories. Many so called healthy foods have excess calories and must be utilized to a minimum during dieting and maintenance programs. Polyunsaturated oils though have health benefits, a mere one ounce contains over one hundred calories. Just like any other food calories must be reduced in order for weight loss to occur.

Q) Do liquid calories count in the over all structure of the diet?

A) Liquid calories must be taken into account when considering the total calories in any one twenty four hour period. Many nonalcoholic drinks are so fraught with sugar when ingested weight gain is inevitable. Most fruit juices, nondietetic sodas, so called energy drinks, protein and milk shakes are many of the culprits in today's weight crisis. Please remember that many liquid diet drinks that claim they are complete meals in reality only satiate the dieter for a brief period of time then hunger sets in. Properly selected drinks from the menus will enhanced weight loss. Alcohol is converted into sugar by the body and should be avoided during a diet period.

Q) Can one diet during the week and stop on weekends?

A) You can't negotiate with your body. Part time dieting does not work. Weekend food binging can negate all the weight loss from the prior week.

Q) Will exercise offset a calorie rich diet?

A) Generally no. The chance of burning sufficient calories by exercising to offset a calorie rich diet is between slim and none.

Q) Should I exercise on an empty stomach?

A) Eating a preworkout meal provides the energy necessary to perform the exercises. Workouts where a person has not eaten for many hours could cause the blood sugar to drop substantially. Symptoms such as fatigue and dizziness may occur inhibiting your exercise.

Chapter Seven

How to Read Labels

The distortion in food labeling has reached new levels of misrepresentation. Not only do food labels distort the contained ingredients in many products they outright lie about them. Inaccuracies in labeling are not new. The Food and Drug Administration and the United States Department of Agriculture require that labels on most packaged goods are in a easy readable format. The Nutritional Labeling and Education Act (NLEA) of 1990 is a major piece of legislation to help the consumer wade through the nutrition murk created by the food industry. Unfortunately, anyone reading the tenets of this legislation would have to be mathematically inclined to understand it. Since the government poorly monitors food labels it is always years behind in catching violators of these promulgated rules of food labeling. The clarity in labeling promised by the NLEA does not translate into reality because the law is so complex the food manufacturer can create its own interpretation of the law. This enables them to find clever ways to distort the labeling process. Therefore, the consumer must be vigilant in applying the information contained on food packages. Labels include information on calories per serving, amounts of protein, fat, fiber and sugar within the structure of the food. Vitamin and mineral data are delineated with percentage of daily requirements manufactured into the product. Information concerning fat content as it relates to trans fatty acids and saturated as opposed to unsaturated fats may also be present.

In an attempt to understand how serving size or portions are listed on food packages the study of cereal box information will illustrate how the consumer is being mislead. Remember I never stated that cereal companies were lying about portion sizes. What they have cleverly done is to utilize different serving sizes so comparison among varying products especially within the same brand is more difficult. An explicit example of misrepresentation occurred when a cereal manufacturer advertised a new healthier version of an existing variety. The company simply shuffled the ingredients to give the appearance there was more fiber and less carbs. The end result the calorie content remained the same as the existing variety and the new alignment of ingredients were no more healthy than before. The best dictum still holds true that the "buyer beware" should apply when purchasing food. Many foods marketed as health foods are no more healthy then the foods they claim to replace. Many times the label has been created to be a marquee to falsely advertise their products. So called diet products are nothing more than minor manipulations of common products on the market. A slight reduction is sugar or adding a small amount of additional fiber or protein to give you a sense that the product is healthier allows food manufacturers the right to call something diet when it is not. The words diet or dietetic are misnomers and should not be used. This variety of food simply does not exist.

Do not be deceived by something called organic. Anything grown in the ground can be considered organic in nature. When a label states it is organic it means the food you are purchasing was farmed in a very specific manner. First and foremost organic farmers fertilize with manure or compost instead of chemicals to promote plant growth. Secondly, organic farmers use neither insecticides nor herbicides in their fields. To rid the crops of insects they might use birds or insect predators to reduce harmful insect invasions. For weed control the organic farmer may rotate crops, till the weeds out of the field or mulch. The organic farmer never gives his animals growth hormone or other chemicals to promote growth or prevent disease. The United States Department of Agriculture has specific requirements for food to be labeled organic. Unfortunately, the monitoring system by this department has been less than adequate so it is your responsibility to check to make sure you are getting organic when it states so. There is no evidence that organically raised foods are more nutritious than conventional products nor is the quality any better than the food it claims to replace. For our diet foods that are not "organic in nature" are more than adequate to achieve your dietary goals.

The first item on the product that catches most peoples' attention is its weight. A simple enough concept. But one only needs to open the box or can and the concept takes on an unreality. The cereal box that looks quite large is less than two thirds full. Or that can of carrots that is half water. Even if the product states weight by volume beware the container makes you think there is a larger amount of product than is actually present.

When you are reading the nutrition label the first thing you encounter is the serving size. This is determined by the food manufacturer based on government guidelines and is supposed to reflect the amount of food generally eaten at one time. This is a very elusive concept. There is no uniformity in the serving size from company to company nor many times within the same manufacturer. All nutritional information on the package label is based on the serving size. A cup of soup maybe an adequate amount for a 110 pound female. But to a 200 pound male a bowl might be a more adequate portion. Two crackers are considered a serving size by most manufacturers but they never state who is eating this so called serving. The number of servings per container denotes how many serving sizes are in a whole package. Foods that are labeled diet or reduced calories are intrinsically misleading by the serving size. The manufacturer only has to reduce the serving or portion size within the product group they are selling. Then they can advertise it as "lower calorie per serving size." A number of Federal laws have been enacted to protect us from illegitimate food claims. The sad fact is Federal monitoring is lax. There are so many ridiculous food product claims it is left to the purchaser to discern reality from fiction.

For the dieter the serving size is very important because it dictates the amount of calories you will eat. This obvious fact is not always obvious when attempting to compare products. Serving size is usually represented by familiar units such as cups, bowls or pieces. One manufacturer may use cups another bowels so comparison shopping is made more difficult. Increasing the confusion even further some companies may print their weights utilizing the metric system. The serving size influences the number of calories and nutrients you might be ingesting so vigilance in comparison shopping is a must. With the complexity noted above utilize the number of calories as your guide instead of the serving size. It will give you a better grasp on how much you will be eating.

Portion control is one of the most difficult tasks the prospective dieter faces. With the ambigous nature of the serving size purported by the food industry a level of confusion is introduced because standardization among product lines is lacking. The effective basis for hundreds of diets presently marketed is a reduction in calories through portion control. By marketing products that utilize various serving sizes the food industry can easily undermine a weight reduction program. Fat content is an example how this can work. When two competing products of a similar nature are marketed claiming reduced fats, the clever company simply reduces the portion size to get the competitive edge. Smaller portions reflect less fat grams in their products and are sold as low calorie food alternatives. Many manufacturers keep the consumer guessing whether they are ingesting saturated or unsaturated fats. Adding in the fact that serving sizes vary among similar products represented by different manufacturers the dieter has a major conundrum to over come. Following the menus in this diet will help you get beyond the food industry's never ending desire to confuse the consumer and purchase less than healthy foods.

The next category to consider is the percentage of nutrients that someone should ingest in any one twenty four hour period. It may be listed as percent daily value, percent recommended daily or recommended daily intake. These recommended nutrients are usually based on a 2000 calorie diet and are in excess of what a dieter should be ingesting. These percentages are based on one portion size. A 15% value across from a nutrient means it meets that percentage of recommend daily allowance for that nutrient. When you see total fat grams and a value of 15% across from it, this means that the food in question meets that percentage of the total allowed fat for the day. Data on percent saturated fat and trans fat may also be listed. Saturated fat should account for less than twenty percent of total fat calories per day as noted by most nutritionists. We recommend minimum to none. Trans fatty acids should never be ingested. Both of these fats can cause heart disease which makes avoidance even more imperative.

Cholesterol is usually listed with the fat information. It is measured in milligrams. This information is useful for those who must observe their cholesterol intake. Most cholesterol the body requires is manufactured by the liver so there is no need to eat much in your diet. Many products such as dairy, meats and eggs all contribute to the blood level of cholesterol. The average American diet is fraught with cholesterol causing an increased incidence in heart disease in younger age groups. There is no specific recommendation for daily cholesterol intake. I recommend as little as possible. Caution must be taken with fresh foods specifically meats which do not delineate cholesterol contents on their labels. People with elevated cholesterol should veer away from these products if they are known to be laden with heavy quantities of fat.

Sodium intake is usually displayed as a percentage of recommended daily value. This is a very important number because many people with vascular disease, hypertension and heart disease must not ingest high quantities of sodium. The recommendations for sodium have been revised downwards over the last decade. Many nutritionists recommmed four thousand milligrams of sodium or less. Some would like to see a daily sodium intake at the two thousand milligram level. For those on a salt restricted diet remember to adjust your sodium intake based on the number of serving sizes you are ingesting.

Total carbohydrates are listed on the box in grams. This category of food is broken down into sugar and dietary fiber. Fiber gives the dieter a quick feeling of satiation with little or no calories. It promotes regular bowel movements and may help reduce cholesterol. Fiber is an essential element of any diet. Sugar is a generic word for many different products. Labels do not present amounts of specific sugar types. Some names for added sugar are high fructose corn syrup, corn syrup, fruit juice concentrate, maltose, sucrose, dextrose, honey and maple syrup. In plain yogurt the quantity of sugar noted on the label comes from the naturally occurring sugar lactose. Yogurt that contains fruit byproducts or what appears to be jelly has two or more times the caloric contents of its plain counterpart. Cereal is a second example of food manufacturers ceaseless desire to overload our systems with sugar. Many of the popular brands contain more than ninety percent carbohydrates. Some food processors do not feel this is enough carbs so they also coat the cereal with sugar increasing the carb contents closer to 100%. When the label says white flour they mean sugar, when they say destrose, maltose, dextran, corn syrup, high fructose corn syrup they mean sugar. The label is an excellent source of information regarding carbs but it fails to delineate how much of each of these sugars are contained in their products. A point to remember white flour, white rice, pasta, potatoes are all examples of food products that mainly breakdown to sugar. Most labels fail to denote what percentage of the days allowance of carbs you are ingesting, for good reasons. First, many people may refrain from purchasing their products due to the excess carbs present. Secondly, most manufacturers use a base diet that is well in excess of any caloric requirements the body needs, therefore determining carb content of a product has very little meaning under these circumstances.

Protein is noted on most labels in grams. There are numerous formulas to denote how much protein is required in different age groups and in specific health conditions. For the dieter it is neither feasible nor practical to calculate protein totals. It is generally recommended that approximately 20 to 30 percent of the diet should be from protein. The Millenium

Diet leans towards the latter number. Protein is utilized in nearly every system of the human body. If the body receives insufficient fats or sugars it can burn protein. The present diet contains sufficient protein to provide safe expeditious weight loss. The label usually states the most minimum information concerning protein.

The last major category enumerated on the label is vitamins and minerals. These are either naturally occurring or added for nutritional enhancement. Vitamins and minerals are listed in percentages of daily requirements. But they are not specific by gender, weight class, age or activity level. Most processed foods have minimal amounts of these nutrients. The labels on cereal boxes display how food manufactures provide misinformation to the public. Most cereals have so much sugar in its different formats that one would think they are eating a candy bar instead. The audacity of these companies to advertise their cereals as healthy especially for children is a gross mischaracterization of their product lines. The negligible amount of vitamins in most of these cereals does not compensate for the tremedous amount of sugar manufactured into them. The list of vitamins will vary depending on the nature of the food. Negligible or trace nutrients are usually not listed. Along with vitamins, minerals such as calcium and iron are listed as percentages of daily requirements. It is a rare label that lists more than two supplements. The bottom line is that the food product is not worth purchasing just for the vitamins.

The Food and Drug Administration (FDA) has strict regulations for label statements such as low "fat" or "low sodium." Unfortunately, the FDA has very few inspectors to review the thousands of products on the market to verify labels. The following definitions will help guide you through the complexity of manufacturers designations. It is presented in an easily readable format in the table below.

STATEMENT ON LABEL	CONTENTS IN ONE SERVING
Calorie free	Less than five calories
Sugar free	Less than 0.5 grams of sugar.
FAT	
Fat free	Less than 0.5 grams of fat
Low fat	3 grams of fat or less
Reduced fat or less fat	At least 25% less fat than regular product
Low in saturated fats	1 gram of saturated fat or less, with no more than 15% of the calories coming from saturated fat
Lean	Less than 10 grams of fat, less than 4 grams of saturated fat and less than 95 milligrams of cholesterol
Extra Lean	Less than 5 grams of fat, 2grams of saturated fat and 95 milligrams of cholesterol
Light (lite)	At least 1/3 fewer calories or no more than half the fat of the regular product
CHOLESTEROL	
Cholesterol Free	Less than 2 milligrams of cholesterol and 2 grams or less of saturated fat

| Lower Cholesterol | 20 or fewer milligrams of cholesterol and 2 grams or less of saturated fat |
| Reduced Cholesterol | At least 25% less cholesterol than the regular product and 2 grams or less of the saturated product |

SODIUM

Sodium Free or No Sodium	Less than 5 milligrams of sodium and no sodium chloride in the ingredients
Very Low Sodium	35 milligrams or less of sodium
Low Sodium	140 milligrams or less of sodium
Reduced Sodium	At least 25% or less sodium than the the regular product

FIBER

| High Fiber | 5 grams or more of fiber |
| Good Source of Fiber | 2.5 to 4.9 grams of fiber |

The above cited table allows the consumer more intuitive choices. You will find that many products make claims of low salt on the front panel but the label on the side panel does not concur. To many foods are labeled whole grains, fruits or vegetables when only token amounts are contained in the product. The shear number of products that are shamelessly mislabeled are staggering. The following misrepresentations were reported by the Attorney General for Connecticutt several years ago during a conference in Washington D.C. to illustrate misleading labels:

1) Fruit Juice Snacks - The package is decorated with pictures of oranges, cherries and strawberries, but the leading ingredients are corn syrup and sugar.

2) Carrot Cake Mix- The box depicts carrots but the only ingredient is carrot power.

3) 100% Fruit Jelly - The strawberry version of "100% fruit" contains only 30% strawberries. The blueberry version contains 43% blueberries. Both have fruit syrup derived from less expensive apple, pineapple or pear juice concentrates.

4) Nutri Grain Pancakes - The label notes the product is made with whole wheat and whole grain. In actuality these pancakes are made primarily from white flour and have more high fructose corn syrup than whole wheat or other whole grain types.

The Connecticutt Attorney General is trying to effectuate change in labeling by pointing out these misrepresentations. I eliminated the brand names because the problem is not contained within any one company. But these illustrations stand by themselves. Competition with certain product classes is keen. The incentive to create labels that bend the truth is out there and the informed consumer will be ahead of the game with the knowledge contained within these pages.

CHAPTER EIGHT

Appetite Suppressants

There is a hugh market for appetite suppressants both by prescription and nonprescription. Unfortunately, prescription appetite suppressants have been the subject of disinformation and junk science by those who know minimal to nothing about them. Those who are in the legal profession both in and outside the government have made it increasingly difficult for physicians to dispense these medications. Patients who utilize low doses of these drugs note a mild to moderate suppression of their appetites. This enables them to lose weight in a more comfortable setting. There is a plethora of data to support their efficacy. The government has made arbitrary determinations that these drugs should not be used for prolonged periods of time without any evidence to support their claims. The legal profession has seized upon these false claims and sued physicians for billions of dollars. Lawyers who represent the government's interests have censured physicians for not following procedures derived from their junk science experts. Preventative medical procedures are a low priority for a government who collects billions of dollars a year from revenues generated by the healthcare industry. When the government visualizes someone who is obese it sees dollar signs. Why rock the boat. Stop the drugs and there are more obese individuals with their various illnesses. It is a win-win situation for the government and the heathcare monopoly. While these drugs are still legal and there are physicians who responsibly prescribe them these pharmaceuticals can be a great asset in the weight loss equation.

There are less than a dozen prescription appetite suppressants. The nonprescription suppressants number in the dozens. This does not include the ones taken off the market for fraudulent claims. For nonprescription varieties the claims of major weight are loss are only noted in anecdotal tales not regulated studies. Within the prescription medication group studies display their efficacy. The dieter must remember none of these drugs burn any calories even if they claim to do so. It is the diet and the diet only that causes the weight loss. The legitimate appetite suppressant should do exactly what it states suppress your appetite. The dose should be the lowest possible to cause the least number of side effects. Whichever type you try know the side effects and how it may affect your health. Those who have health issues should always check with their physician before starting these drugs. This chapter will enumerate the prescription drugs first including their side effects, how they work, what you can expect in terms of appetite suppression and weight loss. The discussions below represent the most common side effects seen. Within this class of drugs there are also many rare side effects that can be encountered. Always read the package insert before starting any of these medications. The following list are some of the more popular prescription diet medications.

1) <u>Phentermine</u> is the most popular prescription diet pill on the market. It provides a mild to moderate suppression at doses of 15mg to 75mg. It has been in existence for at least five decades and in that time period millions of people utilizing Phentermine have successfully lost weight. It works by altering chemicals in the central brain. It is a class four narcotic derivative similar to

amphetamines. It is mildly addicting at dosages much higher than is needed to give adequate appetite suppression. It is metabolized in the liver and excreted in the urine. For those who require a work, school or an insurance physical Phentermine will show up in your blood or urine as a narcotic so let the examiner know ahead of time the type of drug you are using. A single thirty milligram dose may work up to fourteen hours. Traces can be found in your system after one week. Always let your physician or dentist know you are taking this drug as it could affect procedures they may have planned for you.

The most common side effects observed with Phentermine is dry mouth. Some people describe it as cotton mouth. This particular side effect does not fade quickly. It may even stay during the course of use. The only solution for the dry mouth is more fluids. The second most common side effect is constipation. It generally occurs several days into the utilization of the drug. The constipation responds to increased fiber, more fluid and the occassional need for a mild stool softener. Upset stomach on initiation of the drug occurs rarely but appears to subside quickly unless an alternate stomach problem exists such as gastritis.

The side effects that must be addressed quickly are those that effect the vascular and pulmonary systems. Cases of rapid heart rate are rare but are described in the medical literature. Heart valve damage is an extremely rare phenomena with this drug. When Phentermine was paired with another drug Fenfluramine (also called Redux or Pondermine, which was banned over a decade ago) heart valve damage was an issue. Fenfluramine was the toxic component of the two drug regimen. Anyone who experiences unexplained shortness of breath should discontinue the drug immediately and call the prescribing doctor. Under no circumstance should you continue this drug if you notice chest pain or palpitations. Caffeine and other cardiac stimulants should be reduced or even eliminated when using Phentermine. Not only do these stimulants increase cardiac and other side effects they may block the effect of these drugs. People with known heart disease should never be prescribed Phentermine.

Sporadic headaches are noted in a few percentage of patients under treatment. Most headaches occur on the lateral aspects of the forehead and are described as brief, usually several hours or less. They usually respond to Tylenol, Motrin or Aleve. Phentermine can trigger a migraine so caution should be taken if you have a medical history of this problem. This drug can increase intraocular pressure and is therefore contraindicated in glaucoma. It may also affect libido in both sexes.

Phentermine may lower the threshhold for seizures. It is not advisable to use if there is a known or suspected history of seizures. All seizure classes are included in this warning. This drug is also known to cause mild anxiety, irritability, mood swings and insomnia. These mild neurological side effects are transient. Anyone with a history of prolonged depression should not take this drug. The side effects of this drug may start several days after initiation or not at all. Patient histories denote a major variance in the onset of side effects.

Phentermine should NEVER be taken while pregnant. It should be stopped sixty days before attempting to conceive a child. While breast feeding a woman should refrain from utilizing this drug. There is no evidence that it affects birth control medications.

Dermatological diagnoses are rare. The most common skin finding is papular eruptions scattered across the face, especially around the bridge of the nose. Urticaria is extremely rare with this drug.

Endocrine side effects include impotence and changes in libido. These effects are rarely seen. Both sexes may experience libido changes. Treatment is to stop the drug or the problem will persist. Insulin requirements for diabetics may change. If you are a diabetic please consult your doctor before using Phentermine.

Caffeine appears to enhance many of the side effects of Phentermine including elevating your blood pressure and heart rate. The neurological side effects such as anxiety and insomnia also appear to be accentuated. Patients that utilize high doses of caffeine usually request elevated doses of Phentermine. Caffeine appears to have an inhibitory effect on this drug and reduction in caffeinated beverages could enhance the drugs suppressive effects. Those who use large doses of caffeine tend not do well on Phentermine or other amphetamine derived diet pills.

Originally approved by the Food and Drug Administration for a twelve weeks, Phentermine has been found to work well beyond this intended guideline. The FDA allows use of a drug for other purposes once it is licensed. High doses are not recommended because rapid tolerance occurs rendering the drug less effective. The use of Phentermine for long term intervals is very common. Dr. Arthur Frank of George Washington University has written a paper denoting its safe use in a small sample of patients for up to ten years for both weight loss and for maintenance. Since obesity is defined as a chronic disease it is appropriate to treat it with medication as we do with other long term conditions.

2) Phendimetrazine is another popular prescription diet medication. It is listed as a class three narcotic meaning it is

slightly more addicting than Phentermine. It's activity level is much shorter than Phentermine requiring more frequent dosing intervals to achieve proper appetite suppression. Its mechanism of action is not dissimilar from other amphetamine derived diet drugs. It works in an area of the brain called the hypothalamus which controls food cravings. The side effects of Phendimetrazine are similar to Phentermine. This drug may not be as popular as Phentermine because of its shorter life span and its increased potential for addiction. Dosing range for Phendimetrazine varies from 35 milligrams to 210 milligrams. Adjusting the dose is sometimes very tricky and is another inducement to use Phentermine. The same cautions and warning noted in the Phentermine section apply to this drug. It will appear in the urine and blood as a narcotic so let the testing party know you are taking this drug. Phendimetrazine has no capacity to burn fat. It should always be used in conjunction with a diet.

3) <u>Diethylproprion</u> is a class four narcotic diet drug. It is mildly addicting at doses larger than are required for appetite suppression. The dosing range is 25 to 100 milligrams. This drug should not be given to anyone with heart disease, severe hypertension, hyperthyroidism, chronic pulmonary disease and those with a known a history of seizures. It is contraindicated during pregnancy or while breast feeding. Certain types of anemia may also be caused by this drug. Diethylproprion is not as popular as Phentermine and Phendimetrazine because it does not suppress appetite to the same extent. A dose of 50 milligrams per day has helped most dieters achieve their weight goals. The drug should be immediately stopped if chest pain or shortness of breath occurs. When the side effects of Phentermine and Phendimetrazine are to intense Diethlyproprion has been utilized to help patients continue their diet programs.

4) <u>Didrex</u> is a class three narcotic diet drug. This drug is more addictive than Phentermine and maybe the reason why it is prescribed infrequently. Didrex is also called Benzphentermine

and as a derivative of Phentermine shares many of the same side effects. It has the potential for respiratory and cardiac side effects. If shortness of breath or chest pain occur during its utilization stop the drug and notify your physician. Anxiety, irritability, mood swings and insomnia are common symptoms. Didrex is not as popular as the former listed drugs because of its addiction qualities and side effect profile.

5) <u>Xenical</u> also called Orlistat, is a non-narcotic prescription medication that blocks the absorption of up to 30% percent of fat consumed. It was recently approved in a non-presciption format called Alli. The drug is best utilized when large amounts of fat are consumed. The drug has some very uncomfortable side effects including stool incontinence, fecal urgency, oily stools and flatulence. It may also block absorption of vitamins A, D, E and K. The better alternative than taking this drug is to reduce your fat consumption.

6) <u>Meridia</u> also called Sibutramine is a class four narcotic appetite suppressant. It is in the same category as Phentermine in terms of addiction potential. Meridia will test positive for a narcotic when a toxicological blood or urine screen is performed. Its maximum dose is 15 milligrams per day. Meridia's weight loss profile has not lived up to its hype. It is very expensive and lower priced pharmaceuticals are available which give much better appetite suppression. It side effect profile is similar to Phentermine and Phendimetrazine. It is contraindicated in numerous disease states including heart and lung disorders. Severe liver and kidney disease also exclude its use. The government has certified this for weight loss and weight maintenance. But this is a farce because so little weight is lost with it that maintenance has no meaning. I do not recommend this drug.

All of the above prescription drugs except for Xenical can be habit forming. The lowest dose possible should always be chosen. Higher doses may accelerate tolerance to these narcotic derivatives and should be avoided. Many patients have a perception that their energy levels are elevated during a course of these medications. A similar phenomena is noted with caffeine. High doses of caffeine tend to mitigate the suppressor effects of narcotic diet medications. In addition, caffeine may intensify many of the side effects of these medications except for Xenical. With this in mind caffeine should be diminished or eliminated during a course of these drugs. ALCOHOL should be avoided while utilizing narcotic appetite suppressants. The mixture can affect mental clarity and reflex time. Driving should be restricted if a combination of alcohol and narcotic appetite suppressants have been consumed.

Nonprescription diet pills have very little proven value except as a psychological boost. The amount and type of ingredients contained in these drugs may not be accurately labeled on their containers. Great caution should be observed when consuming them for this reason. Except for Alli, there are no available legitimate studies to support their efficacy. Side effect profiles can run the gamut from mild to death. If you have any known medical concerns check with your doctor before using them. The propaganda for these drugs can usually be found in all forms of the media. From the late night informercial to radio testimonials, distortion plays well. The media kings know just how to put together packages of misinformation to make these products sound attractive. A typical commercial starts with anecdotal tales of remarkable weight loss. " I lost twenty pounds the first week utilizing this powder which is the entrails of a rattlesnake." Or "I lost three inches off my waist in the first five days consuming this new fungus extract found in a tropical rain forest whose location is known only to a few individuals." There are no published medically peer reviewed studies to support their claims. The formulas for these products appear to be randomly placed ingredients that make no sense. I have yet to find anyone who has used these type of drugs and achieved any significant weight loss. Alli, the nonprescription version of Xenical has not proven itself to be an effective drug within our patient population. Yet, unknown numbers of websites spew their written nonsense for you, the dieter, to buy their pharmaceutical garbage. Many of these drugs come with diets as part of their packaging. It is the diet and only the diet causing the weight loss. The following list of nonprescription appetite suppressants is extensive. There is no data base to support the manufacturers contention that they work. This list was compiled by its authors who are at website www.dietpills. cc/over-the counter-diet-pills.html.

Abgone	Beta 3
Accelis	Biblica
Accuslim	Bioslim
Adenergy	Blaze Xtreme
Advalean	Black Ice
Advantage Weight Loss	Block and Bind
Alli	Blu Impact
Anatril	BodiLene RFC
Anatrim	Body Slim
Anorex	Brazilian Blaze
Aquadrene	Burn3D
Atkins AM Cleanse	Carb Cutter
Atkins Accel	Carb Dynamx
Carb Helper	Cylaris
Carb Intercept	Deep

Carb Spa
Cardio Stack
Cblock
Charge ASF
Cheat and Eat
Cheaters Relief
ChitoGenics
Chitosan
Choice Natural Weight Loss Pill
Citrimax
Colvera
Cortislim
Cortisol Blockers
Cravex
Curvelle
Cuts 11
EPH 833

Ephedrasil
Ephedrine HCL
Ephedrine P57
Ergolean MC
Ergolean AMP
Eroved
Estrin D
Estrodex
Estro Lean
Everslim

Detoxatrim
Dexatrim Max
Dexatrim Results
Diabetisyn
Diatrin H
Diet Carb Block
Diet Fuel
Diet Cheating Caps
Dietrine Carb Blocker
Dymetadrine Xreme
Eat Less
Emagrece Slim
Endurox
Energy Reserve
Enhance CLA
EPH 200
Fat Cutter
Fblock Xtra
Hardcore Fedramine
Fenphendra
Formastat
Formigen
Formula 9
Fyre
Glucofast
Glucolean
Glucopsyll
Gordonix

Excell Now Energy Pill

FahrenHeit

FatAbsorber TDSL

Fat Blocker Plus

Fat Burners for Women

Fat Converter

Herbathin

Hoodia Bites

Hollywood MetaMiracle

Hot Rox

HydroBurn

Hydrox Slim

Hydroxy lean

Isatori MX-LS7

JetFuel

Kaizen Caffeine

Lean Balance

Lean Out

Lean System

Lean Extreme

Lean Fire

Leptopril

Leptoprin

Maculean

Maxadrine

Mega Fat Burner

Mega Green Tea

Megadrine

Green Tea Fat Burner

GuggulEZ100

Guggulbolic Extreme

H57 Hoodia

Herbal Phentermine

HerbaLife

Leptovox

Lipitrex

Lipo 6

Lipocerin

Lipodren

Lipodrene-SR

Lipodrene Xtreme

Lipojuiced

Liponesta

Liporexin

LipoRidPM

LipoSlim System

LipoSpa

LipoTrim

Lipovar 8

Lipovarin

Lipovox

Lipozene

Nitrix

Nophedra

NOS Matrix

NOX3

Meltdown Z-14

MeltRx 24 Ultra

Metabo Speed XXX

Metabolean

Metabolic Tyrolean

Metabolift

Midnight Stallion

Mini Lean

MiracleBurn

Musculean

Myoffeine

Nature's Supercaps

Nite Trim

Phenterprin

Phentirimine

Phire

Pyruvate 1000

QuickFire

RapidSlim SX

Redline

Relacore

Remedilean

Ripped Power

Ripped System

San Slim

Scorch

Nueslim-19

NV Rapid Weight Loss Beauty Pill

l-EZ Appetite Suppressant

l-EZ Carb Suppressor

l-EZ Fat & Carb Blocker

1-EZ Fat Burner

1-EZ Fat Purger

l-EZ Gugu

Oxydrene

PediaLean

PhenterLean HG

Slenderful

Slim Seduction

Slim Stack

Slimage

Slimquick

Slimquick Night

Smart Burn

Solidax ADX

Soma-Slim

Stacker 2

Stacker 3

Stimerex-ES

Subdue

Superdrine RX 10

Suvaril

Serofil

72 Hour Diet Pill

Shredded

Skinny Mini

Tetrazene

Tetrazene ES-50

Thermalean RX

ThermaSlim

Thermics

ThermoDynamX

ThermoGenics Plus

ThermoGenics Plus Quick Start

ThermoGenics Plus Quick Start for Men

ThermoGenics Plus SF

Thermoloid

Thermonex

Thyrin-ATC

ThyroCuts ll

ThyroSlim AM/PM

Thyroid T-3

Thyrotril

Xenedrine Super Hard Core

Xerisan ASA

Xlean

Xpel

Xylestril

Yellow Bullet

Yellow Jacket

T3

Taraxatone

Thyrox

Tight

Total Lean

TriLean

Trimethylean

Trimspa

Triple Lean

Ultra Diet Fuel

Ultra Carb Intercept

Ultra Diet Pep

Vaporize

Venom Hyperdrive 3.0

VeroSlim

Viva Body

Xelerate

Xenadrine EFX

Xenadrine NRG

Zenalean Pro

Zetacap

Zotrin

ZylorinZymelite

Yellow Swarm

Yogaslender

Zalestrim

Zantrex

Any of these drugs that contained ephedrine or its derivatives were banned in 2004. Many of these products may already be off the market. Their ability to cause weight loss is very questionable. The author does not recommend any of these drugs. Adequate information on the safety and efficacy of these medications in most cases simply does not exist.

Chapter Nine

Vitamins and Minerals

Vitamins are nutrients utilized by all systems of the body for maintenance, growth and energy formation. For dieting purposes a metabolic system that runs more efficiently because of these nutrients will enhance weight loss. Some vitamins are made by the body and others must be consumed. A very common question is what are the best brands to purchase. There is no one best brand. Vitamins are required by the body in trace amounts. Some will be stored by the body for future use and the remaining quantities the metabolism discards. We know these nutrients are necessary because certain disease states occur in their absence. Most brands have the recommended daily amounts for each vitamin. Sometimes their mineral contents fall short of amounts the body requires and further supplementation is necessary. Calcium, is an example of this type of deficit. Most Vitamin tablets have minimal amounts of calcium. In many cases less than 10% of the minimum daily requirement. Supplementation then becomes a necessity. Dosing larger than the body requires is called hypervitaminosis. These large doses are not required by the metabolism and may cause illness to those consuming them. The vitamin hucksters are all over the media claiming their supplements are superior. But they can not present any evidence to support their claims. Most multiple vitamins contain what the government notes are Recommended Daily Requirements or Recommended Daily Allowances (RDA). These requirements vary based on age, activity level and medical status. Unfortunately, the government delineations do not address these specific requirements, therefore consult with your medical provider if your needs are greater or less than the RDA. Many of the store brands are made by mainstream companies and are usually the same or similar to their name brand counterparts. There is no data to support that brand names work any better than their generic alternatives.

For vitamins to work they should be taken over a long period of time. There is no research to indicate how long. For most deficiency states a minimum of three months is necessary. Sporadic use of vitamins does little to enhance your health and well being. Newer studies indicate that vitamins not only have disease preventative properties but they also enhance longevity. Cancer, heart disease and other long term illnesses maybe abated or at the minimum abbreviated by their use. The following discussion will denote each vitamin by its use, physical properties, function, as it relates to their presence or absence and metabolism.

Vitamin A

What is Vitamin A?

Vitamin A is a number of compounds that are essential for many metabolic functions in order for us to survive. There are two common forms that are available depending on which source they are extracted, animal or plant. Vitamin A found in food that comes from animal sources is called Preformed Vitamin A. Another form that is found in many fruits and vegetables is called Provitamin A. Preformed Vitamin A is absorbed into our systems as retinol. This is an active form of this vitamin. The Provitamin A which is a carotenoid can be made by the body into a retinol. Beta carotene is the most efficient of the carotenoids to be converted to Vitamin A. Many vitamin supplements note part or all of their Vitamin A comes from Beta Carotene.

What foods contain Vitamin A?

There are many natural sources of Vitamin A, in its various forms, including lemons, sweet potatoes, carrots, spinach, squash, apricots, cantaloupe, mangos, liver, beef, pork, chicken, turkey, fish, eggs, collard greens and broccoli. Many foods are fortified with Vitamin A including breads, cereals and other processed foods. Since this book deals specifically with rapid weight loss in a healthy way many of these choices need to be avoided because of their high caloric content. The best reference is the menu guide in the diet chapter for types and quantities of foods.

What is the function of Vitamin A?

Vitamin A is utilized by the body in all its specialized systems by enabling cell division and cell differentiation, reproduction, growth and replacement of cellular structure for maintenance of these systems. The visual cortex and its complex eye/optic nerve connections depend on these compounds. Vitamin A helps maintain the surface linings in the respiratory, intestinal and urinary systems. The retina of the eye is dependent for replenishment of its surface on this vitamin. Without this vitamin bacteria are able to enter these systems faster and cause infection. Vitamin A's role as an antioxidant has been called into question by recent science articles. Antioxidants protect cell structures from substances called free radicals that are derivatives of oxygen metabolism. These radicals can damage DNA that can cause chronic health problems. Vitamin A has not demonstrated consistent protective effects from these substances.

What is the appropriate dose for me?

The categorization by age, gender and metabolic condition guide us in choosing the Recommended Daily Allowance (RDA). Most authors use the International Units (IU) measure to keep dosing standard or its equivalent in micrograms. A male over 19 years of age requires 900 micrograms or 3000 IU. A female over 19 years of age requires 700 micrograms or 2300 units. Women who are pregnant increase their dose to 770 micrograms or 2565 IU. Fetal Interactions with this vitamin should always be considered therefore check with your doctor before taking this supplement. Lactating females require 1300 micrograms or 4300 units.

What medical conditions occur in the absence of Vitamin A?

Vitamin A deficiency is very common in many less affluent sections of the world. Where malnutrition exists Vitamin A deficiency exists. Up to half million children become visually impaired from this deficiency each year. In America restricted caloric intake causes this deficiency to occur. Excess alcohol also may lead to this problem. When zinc deficiency exists Vitamin A deficits also occur. Zinc is a necessary cofactor in Vitamin A transport across cell wall structures. When zinc deficits occur stored Vitamin A in the liver is harder to obtain for metabolic purposes.

Night blindness also called Nyctalopia occurs early in this deficiency. Without adequate Vitamin A the cornea and the retina can't process light well. The cornea especially becomes very dry. The ancients new that if they ate liver it somehow cured this disease, and they were right. Liver stores large amounts of Vitamin A.

The likelihood of infections increases geometrically in countries where this deficiency occurs. Many childhood infections are acquired through the respiratory tract. The deficiency causes cells lining areas of the respiratory tract to lose their ability to destroy many bacteria and viruses. Pneumonia is therefore common during this time. There is also an increase in diarrhea because the lining of the gastrointestinal tract becomes more prone to infections during a shortage of this vitamin.

People with disease states that interfere with fat absorption are prone to this deficiency because Vitamin A is then inhibited from reaching areas needed. Many inflammatory conditions of the gastrointestinal tract require elevated levels of Vitamin A. Pancreatic disease, Crohn's disease and Celiac disease are just a few of these conditions blocking the absorption of this vitamin.

One form of Vitamin A called beta carotene may increase the incidence of lung cancer in those who smoke cigarettes. Those who did not smoke did not have the higher risk. More studies need to be done to confirm this finding.

The American diet provides sufficient Vitamin A. Those people who want to supplement their diets with a multiple vitamin tablet will find that all the name brands and their generic counterparts have sufficient Vitamin A. Those women who are pregnant should consult their doctors for the proper dosing of this vitamin. Patients with chronic diseases are also advised to do the same.

What are B vitamins?

B vitamins are a group of eight substances required by the body for cellular repair, cellular metabolism and maintenance of bodily systems. They are water soluble allowing them to be absorbed relatively easily under normal body conditions. The body stores B vitamins within the liver for later use. There are eight B vitamins presently recognized. B1 which is Thiamine, B2 which is Riboflavin, B3 which is Niacin and its derivatives, B5 also called Pantothenic Acid, B6 which is Pyridoxine, B7 which is Biotin or Vitamin H, B9 also called Folic Acid and B12 which is Cobalamin.

What foods contain B vitamins?

Thiamine is found in green leafy vegetables, legumes, sweet corn, brown rice, red meats, egg yokes, grains and nuts. Many food products are fortified with B vitamins and their labels may indicate how much. Riboflavin is found in milk, meat, eggs, cheese, whole grains and legumes. Niacin is found in fish, meats, legumes, peanuts, eggs, milk products, potatoes and yeast. Pyridoxine is found in many products including organ meats, brown rice, whole grains, soybeans, fish, butter and liver. B12 is found in liver, milk, poultry, egg yolks and meat. Folic Acid is found in cereals fortified with it, whole grains, liver, yeast and green vegetables. Pantothenic Acid is found in whole grains, cereals, meats and legumes. Biotin is found in mushrooms, egg yolks, yeast, peanuts, cauliflower and beef liver.

What are the functions of the B vitamins?

1) Thiamine is necessary for carbohydrate metabolism turning complex sugars into glucose. It is a cofactor in a number of enzymatic reactions and is involved in the production of neurotransmitters.

2) Riboflavin is a cofactor in the metabolism of proteins, fats and carbohydrates. It is intimately involved in the preservation of skin integrity and mucous membranes, nerve sheaths that surround nerve tissue and replenishment of cell structure in the cornea of the eye. It is also essential as a cofactor to retard the generation of free radicals from oxidative reactions that damage cells.

3) Niacin also called Nicotinic Acid or Nicotinamide is utilized in numerous reactions for maintenance, support and replacement of cell structure. It has important functions in maintaining the structure of the skin. Niacin enhances the integrity of nerve structure and improves gastrointestinal functions. Many oxidative reactions require this B vitamin to be completed.

4) Pyridoxine is essential in the metabolism of fats, proteins and carbohydrates. It is utilized in the production of red blood cells and in reactions involving amino acid metabolism.

5) Vitamin B12 also called Cyanocobalamin can not be absorbed unless a substance produced in the stomach called intrinsic factor binds to it to enable its absorption. Once B12 is absorbed in the small intestine it is used for the processing of carbohyrates, proteins and fats. It is an integral part of the red blood cell metabolism. Replenishment of nerve sheath structures require B12. This vitamin is a cofactor in the generation and maintainance of DNA.

6) Folic Acid is important in the production of hemoglobin for red cell synthesis. It works in conjunction with B12 to synthesize DNA. Protein breakdown also requires this substance. Folic Acid helps maintain proper cardiac function. It is also an essential nutrient in many biochemical reactions throughout the body.

7) Pantothenic Acid is involved in carbohydrate, fat and amino acid metabolism. A substance called Coenzyme A which is factor in many biochemical reactions requires Pantothenic Acid for synthesis.

8) Biotin works in conjunction with other B vitamins to produce its effects. This substance has the abililty to reduce skin scaling.

What occurs when the body is deficient of B vitamins?

A) Thiamine deficiency though rare is seen in those people who use alcohol excessively. Alcohol reduces the absorption of Thiamine in the gastrointestinal tract. As a result of this effect there are a number of disease states that occur from lack of Thiamine. Beriberi is a disease which has components of anemia, muscle wasting, paralysis and muscle spasms is due to a deficiency of this vitamin. Since Thiamine helps in the manufacture of neurotransmitters the lack of this substance causes certain neurological diseases. Wernicke's Encephalopathy which causes lack of coordination and Korsakoff's Psychosis which causes memory dysfunction are both derived from deprivation of Thiamine. Deficits of this nutrient affect the oral cavity by increasing sensitivity to the teeth, gums and buccal mucosa (oral cavity).

B) A deficiency of Riboflavin causes a number of dermatological and inflammatory conditions including seborrheic dermatitis, glossitis and angular cheilosis.

C) Niacin deficiency is the direct cause of a disease called Pellagra which is associated with dermatitis, diarrhea and a certain type of dementia. Decreased Niacin levels are also associated with pain in the oral mucosa and the tongue. During a deficiency of this vitamin the oral cavity and tongue may become bright red. Niacin has been used to lower cholesterol but the dose required may cause skin flushing, pruritis, headaches and nausea. Caution is advised for this use.

D) Pyridoxine deficiency causes a nerve disease that effects coordination, the ability to think clearly and interferes with sleep. Pyridoxine deficits also causes skin diseases not to dissimilar from niacin and riboflavin deficiencies. Astute dentists recognize an inflammation of the tongue, oral mucosa and lips caused by low levels of pyridoxine in the system.

E) B12 deficiency can occur in a number of ways. When the stomach has an inability to manufacture intrinsic factor, a necessary protein to absorb B12, deficiency occurs. Vegetarians may also experience a deficiency by their lack of intake of foods rich in this vitamin. Pernicious anemia is a result of a deficit of this substance. Symptoms of this disease are reduced feeling or numbness in the extremeties, episodic weakness, skin pallor and fevers. A long term consequence of B12 deficiency is spinal chord and brain damage. B12 deficiency may not be evident early in the course of a disease because this vitamin is stored by the body for a relatively longtime.

F) Folic Acid deficiency mirrors many of the symptoms of B12 deficit including anemia, stunted growth, neurological problems and inflammation or irritation of the mouth. Folic Acid is prevalent in many foods. Those with poor diets such as alcoholics, conditions that inhibit food adsorption and those without access to proper diets evolve this deficiency.

G) Pantothenic Acid: There is no known disease state associated with a deficiency of this vitamin.

H) Biotin deficiency causes a type of dermatitis which forms scales and eventually exfoliation of the skin. Egg whites contains a food product called Avidin. This chemical blocks the body's utilization of Biotin. The caveat is is you have to eat an excessive amount of egg whites to get this effect.

The following dosages are utilized when a person does not have a deficiency of any of the B vitamins. The medical literature contains a wide variance in dosing of these vitamins. When a deficiency state is diagnosed by your healthcare practioner the replacement dosages could be many times the normal range. Always read your labels to assure yourself of proper dosing.

B Vitamin	Dosage
Thiamine (B1)	1 to 1.5 milligrams/day
Riboflavin (B2)	1 to 1.8 milligrams/day
Niacin (B3)	extremely variable
Pyridoxine	1.5 to 2.0 milligrams/day
Folic Acid	100 to 400 milligrams/day
B12	extremely variable (2 to 6 micrograms)
Biotin	no standard
Pantothenic Acid	no standard

Vitamin C

What is Vitamin C?

Vitamin C is a water slouble substance which the body can not store because it is rapidly excreted into the urine. It requires a continued replenishment to perform its functions.

What is the function of Vitamin C ?

Vitamin C is required for formation and maintenance of a supporting tissue called collagen. Collagen is found in skin, bone and muscle. Supporting structures of the body including joints replenish their collagen regularly and Vitamin C is a cofactor in its manufacture. Vitamin C also perfoms the functions of an antioxidant by protecting dietary lipids and fat soluble vitamins from oxidation. Some authors believe Vitamin C improves immunity at mega dose levels. This remains in the realm of debate. Without this vitamin wounds would not heal, torn ligaments would not repair themselves and blood vessels would not perform their main functions.

What foods contain Vitamin C?

Vitamin C can be obtained from fresh fruits and vegetables. Some with the highest concentration of this vitamin include citrus fruits (oranges, grapefrutis, lemons, limes), papayas, strawberries, mangos, kiwis, melons, raspberries and cranberries. Vegetables with increased concentrations of Vitamin C include green peppers, broccili, turnips greens, cauliflower, cabbage, carrots, parsley, potatoes, yams, sweet potatoes and onions.

What are the signs of a Vitamin C deficiency?

Vitamin C deficiency affects a multitude of bodily systems. Sailors have known for centuries that prolonged periods without citrus fruit caused their gums and oral mucosa to bleed, wound healing would be impaired and infections would be increased in frequency. These symptoms were classified as a disease called Scurvy. Other symptoms of Vitamin C deficiency include suppression of the immune system resulting in more infections, anemia, swollen joints, poor tooth enamel and slowing of the metabolism which may affect your weight.

What is the appropriate dosage of Vitamin C?

Standard daily dosage for males is 90 milligrams and 75 milligrams for females. During illness or other bodily stress these doses may vary greatly. Some authors recommend doses in the thousands of milligrams range. The efficacy of these megadoses continues to be debated.

Vitamin D

What is Vitamin D?

This is a fat soluble nutrient which the body can manufacture or can be ingested. The body manufactures this chemical by utilizing ultraviolet light to alter chemicals in the skin. In conjunction with the liver and the kidney it becomes activated. There are several forms of Vitamin D. Calciferol is the most active format.

What is the function of Vitamin D?

Vitamin D functions to preserve normal blood levels of calcium and phosphorus by enabling calcium absorption in the intestines. Vitamin D enhances the mineralization of bone improving its strength. Some recent research suggests that Vitamin D may increase longevity, strengthen the immune system and reduce the frequency of certain cancers.

What foods contain Vitamin D?

In the United States many foods have Vitamin D added in the manufacturing process. Milk is supplemented with this vitamin as well as many breakfast cereals. Salmon, Mackeral, tuna in oil and sardines in oil are some other sources.

What occurs during a deficiency of Vitamin D?

Vitamin D also called the "sunshine vitamin" because the skin participates in its manufacture helps prevent a disease called Rickets. With Rickets the bones become weak, brittle and can not maintain their physical shape. People without sufficient sun exposure and/or diets supplemented with Vitamin D are at risk. Immunity from infections may also occur during deficits of this vitamin.

What is the appropriate dose of Vitamin D?

For adults the recommendations vary in the range of 200 to 800 international units per day. In severe deficiency states the dosing exceeds this range into the thousands of units per day. Check with your health professional if the indication for this vitamin is other than standard maintenance.

Vitamin E

What is Vitamin E?

Vitamin E is a group of eight antioxidants. Alpha tocopherol, one of these antioxidants, has the greatest predominace in the human body and in most brands of vitamins.

What is the function of Vitamin E?

The essential function of Vitamin E is to bind up free radicals resulting from oxidation of fatty acids in the body. By performing this function cell membranes which contain these lipids remains intact. This vitamin also affects the immune system by inhibiting certain enzymes that reduce its activity. Another property of Vitamin E is to inhibit platelet aggregation which may prevent strokes and heart disease.

What are the food sources of Vitamin E?

Many food sources contain this vitamin such as olive oil, safflower oil, sunflower oil, almonds, peanuts, spinach, hazel nuts and avocados. Most of these foods are very high in calories. Therefore, supplements have become very popular sources of this vitamin.

What occurs in a deficiency of Vitamin E?

Prolonged Vitamin E deficiency causes a number of neurological symptoms. These include problems with coordination and balance, peripheral nerve disease impairing sensation, retinal damage, loss of strength in muscle structures and immune system dysfunction. Children are especially prone to diseases caused by a deficit of this vitamin.

What is the recommended adult dose?

The dose for adults is 15 to 30 milligrams (23 to 45 international units) of alpha tocopheral per day for someone who has no history of a Vitamin E deficiency. Doses in the hundreds of milligrams may help prevent heart disease and enhance the immune system. Many of these studies have variable results and the best advice would be to wait until more definitive data is in.

Vitamin K

What is Vitamin K?

Vitamin K is a fat soluble substance which is involved in blood clotting. It enables certain enzymes in the clotting cascade to perform their functions. This vitamin is found naturally in certain plants and is manufactured by bacteria in the intestine.

What is the function of Vitamin K?

The complex blood clotting mechanism requires proteins manufactured in the liver. Clotting factors two, seven, nine and ten derived from this organ require this vitamin for their ultimate function. Vitamin K activity is blocked by the anticoagulant Warfarin (Coumadin). This vitamin is essential to the clotting mechanism in a number of key areas to allow the entire system to correctly function. With a deficit of Vitamin K, death do to uncontrolled bleeding may result.

What foods contain Vitamin K?

Broccoli, kale, lettuce and spinach contain this vitamin. It can also be found in numerous oils such as canola, soybean and olive. Bacteria in the intestines are also a major source Vitamin K.

What happens in a deficiency of Vitamin K?

In Vitamin K deficiency some of the manifestations are ease of bruising, nosebleeds, prolonged bleeding from a cut, blood in the stools, bleeding gums and excessive menstrual bleeding. This deficiency occurs rarely because of the body's access to this vitamin through foods, supplements and internal synthesis of this substance.

What is the appropriate daily adult dosage of Vitamin K?

There is no recommended daily allowance for Vitamin K. Instead, the categorization of adequate intake is established based on the food ingestion of healthy individuals. Daily doses for men are 120 micrograms and for females it is 90 micrograms. Since the body also manufactures Vitamin K adequate dosing amounts have yet to be derived.

MINERALS

Minerals are elements or compounds that the body requires in trace amounts to perform its organic functions. Many of these substances work in conjunction with one another to maintain the body's homeostasis. Every system of the body requires these minerals. The most common minerals utilized by the body are delineated below.

CHROMIUM

This mineral has had much hype concerning its ability to enhance weight loss. There is no proof of this. Chromium works with insulin to metabolize glucose. It may also lower cholesterol to reduce the incidence of plaque formation. As a weight loss supplement it simply has not proven effective.

IRON

Most of the body's iron is utilized to manufacture red cells. Its unique interaction with the heme molecule allows oxygen to be carried by these cells to the tissue level where it is released. Deficiency of iron causes fatigue, anemia and neurological disease such as learning disorders. A prolonged deficiency may affect the immune system. It has no known appetite suppressant effects.

MAGNESIUM

Magnesium is a cofactor in many enzymatic reactions affecting most bodily systems. In muscle metabolism and cardiac function its presence is essential. It enables hormones and enzymes to perform their functions efficiently. Some studies suggest it may reduce plaque formation in arteries. Magnesium influences nerve signal transmission and may improve memory and other higher brain functions.

CALCIUM

Calcium is a cofactor in reactions involving nerve conduction and muscle contraction. By virture of these two uses Calcium affects every organ system in the human body. The heart muscle requires Calcium to contract. Nerve structure could not move information throughout the body without this mineral. Strong bones require an adequate supply for maintenance and growth. Blood clotting would be less efficient in a Calcium reduced environment. Multiple vitamins never contain enough Calcium. Supplementation is usually required with a dosing of 1000 to 1500 milligrams per day.

SELENIUM

Selenium has many functions in the human body. It has both antioxidant and anti-inflammatory properties. It purportedly can reduce the incidence of cancers of the prostate, breast and the intestines. Its ability to enhance the immune system could be the basis for its anti-cancer properties. Some studies suggest that along with other nutrients it reduces the chances of dementia specifically Alzheimer's Disease. Dosage range is 200 to 400 micrograms per day.

PHOSPHORUS

Phosphorus is utilized in many chemical reactions throughout the body from preserving muscle integrity and enabling muscle contraction to bone maintenance and growth. Calcium and Phosphorus work in conjunction to build bone matrix. Phosphorus is an integral factor in the flitration process in the kidney. Daily dosing varies between 800 to 1200 milligrams.

ZINC

The ubiquitous nature of this mineral in the body is reflected in the numerous systems it is chemically involved. Insulin requires zinc to perform its functions. Testosterone levels are diminished when there is a deficiency of this mineral. Red cell production and the immune system depend on this element in trace amounts. Its antioxidant properties may reduce infections. Daily dosing varies from 10 to 25 milligrams.

About the Author

The author, Mark Davis M.D., a native of New York City, graduated from the State University of New York at Syracuse with a doctoral degree in Medicine in 1978. For the last twelve years his medical practice has been devoted entirely to weight reduction and nutrition. The Millenium Diet, The Practical Guide For Rapid Weight Loss evolved by studying the diet histories of thousands of patients and the results are consolidated into this unique program.

For lecture requests or questions about this book the author can be reached at the following email address: MILLENIUMDIET@GMAIL.COM. To purchase a copy of this book the email address is WWW.MILLENIUMDIET.COM.

Made in the USA
Monee, IL
07 July 2026